YOUR CONCISE GUIDE TO THE MEANING
OF LIFE

Your concise guide to the meaning of life

STEPHAN DE JONGHE

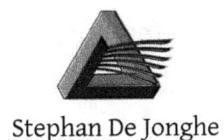

Stephan De Jonghe

Welcome to

Your Concise Guide to the
Meaning of Life.

Well, at least as the concept is understood by this author.

> *Quote: The body is an amazing input-output system. It absorbs and it purges.*
> *Your mind, however, has the wonderful capacity to create more than it consumes.*
> *All of us should learn to use it more efficiently, and thereby reap the benefits.*
> *Stephan De Jonghe*

> *Quote: Life is too precious to waste it on only doing the mundane.*
> *Stephan De Jonghe*

Special thanks to my lovely wife – Deb. Her support, suggestions, and input are always both invaluable and appreciated.

Thank you to my neighbour - Ashley, a good friend, a proof-reader, and a person who openly encourages my writing.

Thanks to my daughter Monique. Her suggestions are always appreciated and respected.

Copyright © 2023 by Stephan De Jonghe
ABN: 84369678327

All rights reserved. No part of this publication may be reproduced, distributed, or transmitted, in any form or by any means, including photocopying, recording, or other electronic or mechanical methods, without the prior written permission of the author, except in the case of brief quotations embodied in critical reviews and certain other non-commercial uses permitted by copyright law.

For permission requests, write to the publisher at: stephansfolliclefarm@gmail.com

Ordering Information: Special discounts are available on quantity purchases by corporations, associations, and others. For details, contact the publisher at the email address above.

ISBN 978-0-6453718-2-6 (paperback)
ISBN 978-0-6453718-3-3 (e-book)
USA
ISBN 0645371823 (paperback)
ISBN 0645371831 (e-book)

Contents

1 Introduction
2 My other book
3 What is the concise meaning of your life.
4 Families and healthy communication.
5 Our need to belong.
6 Giving and receiving.
7 How constructive is your criticism?
8 Self-determinism and what it can do for you.
9 Faith and how to use it to your advantage.
10 Fate and why we need to understand the concept.
11 Our need for affirmation.
12 Why the world seems to be a worse place to live on than it actually is.
13 Five emotions you should learn to minimise.
14 Acute stress responses and hyperarousal. What does it actually mean?
15 Let us take a look at high achievers.
16 Where are you emotionally?
17 How to reduce emotional stress and why this is a good thing.
18 Six important questions you need to answer about everything you do.
19 Why we should understand the Law, Ethics, Morals, and Values.
20 Why it is good to feel pride and to be proud of your skills and achievements.
21 Why we should understand needs, wants, want to, and have to.
22 The decision-making process.
23 The end of your life, and the end of this book.
About the author - I know him well.

~ 1 ~

INTRODUCTION.

> **Warning:** If this book reads to you like as if I'm giving you a lecture, then that's probably true. My aim is to teach you my suggestions on how you can improve your life. This will be just like me giving you Castor Oil by the dessert spoon. It is far easier for me to dispense than it'll be for you to swallow, but by doing so we should be able to unblock your mind. My goal is to give you some benefit - Stephan De Jonghe

> Quote - With some people you only need to point out the remedy: with most others, they'll need to have it rammed into them. - Seneca - A Stoic Philosopher.

For all of my adult years, I have been interested in philosophy, sociology, psychology, and history. I've eagerly read books by inspiring authors, and I have, slowly, over the decades, formed opinions on what life is all about. I often joked that one day I'll achieve ultimate wisdom, and then take all that understanding to my grave. But no, that's not true, as I've always intended to share my views, and opinions, on the meaning of life for the possible benefit of others. Writing and publishing this book is the easiest way for me to achieve that.

When I told my daughter that I was writing this book, she replied. "Yes, I can believe you'd be doing something like that. I look forward to reading it".

There are many books written on how to improve your health, diet, exercise, state of mental health, and longevity. I've tried my best not to write just another one of those books. They are great reads and when combined they have useful advice. You should research them and glean as much useful knowledge from them that you can. I have been doing this all my adult life, so I now recommend that you do so also. I've often felt that many of these books failed to cover some of the reasons why we needed them in the first place. In this book, I'll do my best to fill that gap.

We need to better understand the nature of common human problems, so we can focus on the optimal solution path and properly deal with them.

Okay. Let's begin with some heavy stuff. These four areas of study might seem simple enough, but they are actually very complex. They are also highly compatible, and for you to truly gain an insight into the meaning of your life, you should continuously study them as they'll give you constant benefit.

Philosophy

Philosophy is easily defined as the study of the nature of knowledge, learning, and the continual obtainment of wisdom. The practitioner delves into the question of reality and of existence. They attempt to learn about themselves and their interactions with others. They also gain understanding about how they are seen by others, and how others interact with them. I suggest you become a student of philosophy.

You may never truly master it, but wow, the view along the journey is magnificent. I consider myself as an individual that is practicing Stoicism as my preferred philosophy. This is the mindset of being virtuous about everything, all the time.

Stoics believe that destructive emotions lead to errors in judgment, and so they tend to remain calm in a crisis. Stoics', much like Buddhist, believe in eliminating negative emotions and negative outcomes. Their objective is to control their own pleasures, emotions, and desires, by curbing their egos.

Stoic's judge a person more about their behaviour, and less about their words. Actions will always speak louder than words.

> Quote - Well done is better than well said. - Benjamin Franklin.

Sociology

Sociology is the study of how a society develops, its structure, and how it functions. It examines the evolution of its problems and examines their causes and importantly, their remedies. By developing a greater understanding of your own society, you can better prepare for its challenges, and therefore capitalise on its opportunities.

Psychology

Psychology is the study of the human mind and all of its functions. It looks at behaviour as an individual, as a couple, and as a group. It also studies the effects on an individual, couples, and groups that are intermingling, or working with, other individuals, couples or groups. I also suggest you become a student of psychology. Even as a student you will benefit from a greater understanding of yours and others behaviour.

History

The study of past events and how they shaped our modern world helps you to understand why things are the way they are and hopefully we can avoid repeating the mistakes of the past. It will also help gain an insight into where we as a society are heading.

> *Tip - Be careful about sharing your knowledge with others or falling into the trap of helping others before you've helped yourself. Don't become one of those people that mean well, but give inappropriate, unqualified, and often irrelevant, advice. (Hopefully, I'm not now one of those people, as that would be ironic). This book therefore is for your benefit, so use it to tailor your personal journey with the aim to giving yourself and your life, greater meaning. If you do want to help others, be sure to only offer suggestions or ideas and avoid making them sound like instructions.*

Consider the following thought.

A group of people are highly predictable, but an individual person is highly unpredictable.

Many people consider this to be an accurate comment on human nature. Groups tend to behave in predictable patterns. Small study groups accurately predict events like elections, fashion trends, music, art, and gastronomic sensations.

When examining the individual, it would appear to be harder to predict what they'll choose to do. This is because all individuals are faced with options. The outcome is determined by which option they'll choose. Black or white, up or down, left or right. When they are faced with two options, we have a fifty percent chance of correctly estimating which one they'll choose. The more options, or independent variables there are, the lower the odds of us accurately predicting the outcome, and hence they are thought to be unpredictable.

The reality is that as individuals, we need others to be predictable, this is particularly true when they are driving a car. We want our life partners to be predictable, and our bosses and mentors to be very predictable. As a child, our parents or guardians demanded that we were predictable. They may even have engaged some form of retribution, or punishment, when our unpredictability caused them stress or financial hardship. As a small child we needed our parents and guardians to be predictable. We were read the same books, and watched our favourite movies, or television shows, because they felt safe and comforting. We may like the idea of being surprised, or being spontaneous, but few of us truly are. We learned from a young age and painful experiences that when an unpredictable behaviour backfires, the result can be mutually devastating.

Marketers depend on our predictability. It's how they map out the optimal way to supply goods and services to their consumers.

Political parties vying to win elections want predictability and Governments need predictability to be able to provide the correct mix of services to the people of their country. They don't always get it right, but we expect them to be making informed decisions based on our predicable needs.

Much of our enjoyment of life comes from matching our reality to our expectations. Predictable people tend to enjoy life more because their expectations are more easily satisfied. Innovation and change are only tolerated in small steps. Study history to learn that this is true.

> *Observation - A busy traffic intersection and the traffic management lights are not working. Instead of confusion and accidents, motorists work together, using nonverbal communication, to take turns and keep the traffic flowing in all directions. Everyone understands the need to work together, and everyone gets safely through the intersection. By behaving in a predictable manner, we continue to make progress.*

~ 2 ~

MY OTHER BOOK

> *Quote - It is okay to have multiple personalities', as long as they are orderly, polite, collaborative, and well groomed. - Stephan De Jonghe*

In my fiction novel "Follicle Farm – A Novel adventure," I introduced Bobby, a Mitochondria Follicle Farmer who was ambitious enough to rise through the ranks to become a Quality Control Manager for human hair growth in the person in which he resides. He and his assistant Banjo, explore and learn about some of the functions of the human body. Bobby's comedic experiences included interactions with Mind Managers.

So, who are our Mind Managers? Mind Managers are human cells that are responsible for all human thought and behaviour. Each mind manager has a team of assistants to help them research, plot, devise, and persuade the benefits of their department's intentions for human behaviour to the other mind managers. They are separated into two main categories, voting and non-voting. A voting manager gets to participate in debating what their human will actually say and do. A non-voting manager has thoughts and plans, but only a voting manager can arrange for them to be implemented.

It is all very complex, and no-one knows for sure exactly how many mind managers there are as their numbers are constantly increasing, and their roles tend to evolve as their human grows older.

Excerpt from the book – Follicle Farm – A novel adventure

> *Bobby took a deep breath. 'What does the mind actually do?' he asked hoping not to sound impertinent.*
>
> *'What do you think we do?' Jeremiah was curious.*
>
> *Jeremiah indicated that they should sit, and they both did so. The bag took on Bobby's shape and he was instantly comfortable.*
>
> *'Gather information, talk about problems, make decisions and issue directives...,' Bobby answered hopefully.*
>
> *'It's more than that...,' Jeremiah explained patiently. 'The official textbook version goes like this, "the mind actively processes the flow of information, through elementary drives and complex motives to set out important information about reality. It relates bits of information, synthesises them to construct plans and programs of behaviour. These are expressed by vocalising thoughts or by transmission of these thoughts into action throughout the body."*
>
> *'Wow,' Bobby was impressed. At least he thought it sounded impressive. He wished he understood what it meant.*

You can learn more about the world of Follicle Farm at my website www.folliclefarm.com.au.

~ 3 ~

WHAT IS THE CONCISE MEANING OF YOUR LIFE?

The abridged answer to that question is.... "You are alive to do". A more detailed explanation is that "You're here to do... things".

A now for the clincher – The greatest achievement that you can aspire to, is to give your life significant meaning.

Now, let that soak in.

You could go as far to say that your life is doing a list of verbs. The important aspect is to choose them wisely, ensure they are compatible, do them enthusiastically and gain both pleasure and benefit from them, and whenever possible, to do so with others.

That's it. You have it. You now know the answer and so you can now close this book and go off and do meaningful things.

Cheers and good luck.

> Quote - *If you want to know what the next five years of your life will be like, look at the past five. The only way for life to change is for you to change.* Jim Rohn

Okay. You didn't close the book. You must be curious about what comes next. You're investing more time reading this because you want extra value from this book. Possibly, you're looking for a change in how you are managing your life and you want to improve it.

Good for you.

At the most basic level of life, we have a beating heart to circulate our blood, we're inhaling air, we're consuming and digesting food, and importantly, we're eliminating waste to make room to do it all again. Dead people don't do these things.

You can easily extrapolate that the human body constantly completes numerous functions. The Medulla Oblongata is located in the brain stem, and it regulates all those automated functions so that we don't have to spend time thinking about them. Imagine it as a massive room with thousands of workers monitoring screens that show everything from heart rates, blood flows, urine levels, and breathing. They receive and disseminate billions of messages which they categorise, analyse, understand, and they react as required.

We must sleep as doing without is not an option. What is an option is where we choose to sleep, and who accompanies us when we do sleep (or try to). We have choices to make about what we wear, the type of surface we rest on, what coverings we use. We can choose to have our sleep interrupted artificially at a pre-set time.

We must eat and drink. We can't live without doing so. We do have choices about what we consume. These range from the basic requirements for life, to the full culinary and gastronomic experiences. Our choice is restricted to our current accessibility, affordability, and personal preferences. Remember GIGO. Garbage In leads to Garbage Out. A diet defines what you eat. Select the foods that give you both nutritional benefit and pleasure in quantities that are sufficient to sustain you. This is very well documented, and you should research other books to learn more. The only major roadblock to successfully managing your optimal diet is will power. To achieve this level of control you'll need to master the programming of your own mind and I'll discuss this in greater detail later in the book.

We must move. Doing some exercise will produce immediate benefits. Being active gives us energy. Only sit and rest for as long as it is required to recharge the body. Movement is always beneficial and structured movement through enjoyable exercise, whatever form it takes, will increase your happiness. This is well documented, so do the research and learn the benefits. The only major roadblock to successfully managing your exercise is your own lack of will power.

We must have shelter and clothing. Without these we would be exposed to the elements, and that would seriously diminish the quality of our life. It would also shorten our lifespan. Again, we have choices which are only restricted by our current accessibility, affordability, and personal preferences.

We must learn. Without learning we are doomed to be totally dependent. Just as a newborn baby, we must grow our bodies and our minds. To grow muscle tissue, we must exert effort and stretch our muscles. To increase our knowledge and understanding, we must stretch our minds. Always be learning. By improving your mind, and your body, you'll give your life more meaning which improves your happiness. Confidence is the best cure for stress.

> Quote -
> If you are thinking a year ahead, plant seeds.
> If you are thinking ten years ahead, plant a tree.
> If you are thinking one hundred years ahead, educate the people.
> From Kuan Tzu - a repository of early Chinese thought.

Whilst learning about how to improve our sleeping, eating, drinking, movement, sheltering, and clothing options, we have a massive scope to achieving more of what we desire. I'll show you how later in this book. My desire is to offer you my suggestions on **how you can become the person you want to be.**

> Quote - There is no point in running away in your own company.
> - Seneca

You've already read that to be alive is to do things. It is this act of doing, however minor, that sets you apart from dead people.

Humans have an enormous capacity for achievement. They invent things that enhances their lives and others around them. They sell and market things, often at a profit. They are artistic, they are performers, carers, cleaners, designers, healers, administrators.... The list is too long to list them all, so consider your occupation, hobbies, interests, and sporting activities, listed here.

The one common denominator that all truly successful people have, is that they took somewhere between nine and eleven years of determined and dedicated study, and practice, to gain the experience to achieve the greatness in their field. Procrastination is the enemy and persistence, despite adversity, will reap deserved rewards.

Humans also have the capacity to love, help, and hope. These forces set the stage for a significant number of activities for us humans to discover, learn, master, adapt, and teach. We are by nature nurturers and carers. Ninety percent of us spend a great deal of our time being a better person for others.

We live in a society that cares, protects, and teaches others. Not just our loved ones, family members, and friends, but also complete strangers. For the most, we desire to advance the human condition. This also gives us choices and so the fuller meaning of life, is to be fully engaged with others in all these choices. We desire to maximise the benefits for ourselves, and those connected, however remotely, around us.

With few exceptions, humans love living in a community. Our village is that of connectivity. If you have any doubts, then consider our use of our mobile phone and our connectivity through various social platforms. Look at our willingness to participate in clubs, sports, and hobbies, where we happily seek out like-minded people to form friendships, relationships, and opportunities.

Quote – To procure friendship for the better and not for the worse is to rob it of all its dignity. Seneca

Side note - Douglas Adams, author of the "Hitchhiker's guide to the galaxy" series, and other novels, wrote that the answer to the ultimate question of the meaning of life, the universe and everything, was **forty-two**. *In his novel, philosophers fed all available information into a super-computer known as Deep Thought. The computer was then asked to determine the answer and after many millennia it determined an ambiguous response.*

When confronted, Deep Thought replied that the problem wasn't in the answer, but in the question.

As a fan of Douglas Adams, along with many millions of other people, Deep thoughts response "forty-two" was adopted as a fun way of dealing with our lack of understanding of the meaning of life.

Now I'm thinking that perhaps Douglas had some subliminal notion of what the true answer is. **Forty-two = For-we-to-do.**

Just a thought.

~ 4 ~

FAMILIES AND HEALTHY COMMUNICATION.

> Ancient proverb - The best things in life, aren't things.

> Quote: Persons engaged in a quarrel, begun by using conversational tones. - Seneca

Have you ever thought of something to do that is fun, desirable, or is important to you or for your family to do, but have failed to communicate it to others, only to learn that another family member announced a similar idea of their own, before you could speak out? We all have, and this is a common source of conflict. It can be that I have it in my mind that we should do this one way, but you have it very differently in yours. It is a very common occurrence amongst spouses, and it happens often in all families. So how do we prevent this from causing an issue or an upset? If you have a plan that includes others, detail those plans to others as soon as you can. Here, procrastination is your enemy. Family plans and family activities always have a wide variety of independent variables. Everyone has an opinion and a desired outcome. The key here, is to get in first.

There are three types of family members.

1. Those that want to be in charge of family activities.
2. Those that want to go with the flow.
3. Those that claim to go with the flow, but actually want to be in charge.

It is the last type that amplify family problems as they are often actively, or innocently, sabotaging the efforts of others by increasing confusion, distrust, and disharmony.

> *Observation - When applied to business, or government, communication shouldn't be such a problem. There are hierarchies, procedures, and protocols, for decision making. Meetings and decision making tends to be formal and there are less opportunities for ambiguity in outcomes. Formal organisations have, or hopefully should have, learned from past mistakes.*

Families, however, can have multiple variables and numerous decision makers. They are therefore a breeding ground for emotional conflict.

We are more comfortable lying to family members than to others. This could be because we feel less threatened by the consequences. We often lie for altruistic reasons, privacy concerns, reduce threats, avoid punishments, and sometimes simply to cope. Some lies are uttered to cause mischief. You can lie to others, but you can't lie to yourself. To increase your credibility, learn to minimize their use.

> Quote: *If you tell the truth, you don't have to remember anything.* Mark Twain.

So how do we negate this negativity and in the process improve the quality of our lives through reduced disappointments? The earliest lessons were learned when we were children.

1. Get in first. If you're planning an event, be the first to secure the date, time, location, and to get those details out to the potential participants as soon as possible.
2. Sound the others out. Gain a consensus. Invite them to participate but be sure not to make it sound like a command.
3. Avoid using intermediaries to communicate your message or invite. Talk directly with those people involved or affected. If there are many in the group, write down the details and then share them out. This is how you get everyone on the same page.
4. Treat all family members and friends with respect.
5. Don't dominate the dialogue. Conversations are about an exchange of ideas and experiences. Encourage the others to speak.
6. Develop your listening skills. Too many people are so focused on what they are planning and what they want to say, that they don't really listen or try to understand the other person.
7. Show enthusiasm. Make the event feel like it is a worthwhile thing to do.
8. Accept graciously, or not at all. Don't thwart others with your own improvements or embellishments, without being invited to do so. You devalue the experience from the host if you are takeover person. (Aside from a health or safety issue). You can offer, but you shouldn't impose.
9. Be mutually beneficial. Help each other in a balanced way. Reciprocate assistance. Users end up becoming losers.

10. Offer praise in proportion to deservedness.
11. When your children think of fairness and integrity, hopefully, they'll think of you.
12. Use humour wisely and appropriate to the situation. I caution against teasing as it can hurt the recipient much more than the perpetrator realises. Consider consequences.
13. Capitulate graciously.
14. Being kind is more important than being right.
15. Give materially and emotionally at a level that you feel comfortable with and receive graciously. The more genuine we are, the greater the value of the act.
16. Offer suggestions, not commands. It is okay to have your own opinions, but you should accept that others may have a different opinion, and that doesn't mean they are wrong, or are against you.
17. It's not a competition unless you agree that it is a competition. Call it when it is, and always be dignified when you are victorious.
18. Don't use family members as free labour. They'll quickly learn to avoid you.
19. Give extra consideration to the very young and the very old. They need your help, and they should reciprocate with their gratitude.
20. Avoid using family members as your "Go to person" when you have personal problems. Circumstances change and often what is said in confidence can be deliberately, or inadvertently revealed to others and this may ruin you. (Also, don't use work colleagues for the same reason)
21. Don't drag up issues, or mistakes, that were made by others in the past. If it is resolved, let it go.
22. Faults of the parents, or siblings, do not automatically become the faults of the others.
23. Accept that people do make mistakes. Judge them for what they do next. If they're sorry, apologetic, and want to make

good, then forgive them. If they try and deny their mistake, despite the evidence against them, or are arrogant and feel they can "Get away with it," because they are family, then you can take it further.
24. Become the person that is capable to forgive and move on, after the issues are resolved.
25. Minimise regrets. They'll weigh heavily on your emotions and slow you down.
26. Don't raise your voice in anger. Disagreements and arguments start as conversations that turn bad. Angry voices elevate the tension and worry others.
27. Honesty is the best policy but use diplomacy and tact. Consider the feelings of others and their sensitivities.
28. Lies imprison the teller.
29. A stalemate can sometimes be resolved by all parties agreeing to forget the problem and move on as if it never happened. This technique does work but it should be the exception and not the rule. Pressing the reset button too often will establish a trend that is both observable and measurable, and ultimately undesirable.
30. Alienate family members only as a last resort. If you are in physical, or mental danger, then you should break away from them. Permanently if you have too.

> Question - What costs you nothing but is invaluable to the receiver?
> Answer - A sincere thank you. Be generous with deserved gratitude.

So why are relationships with families so much harder than they are with friends? The answer is easy. You get to choose your friends.

> *Personal experience – Families are most often about raising children into becoming responsible adults. I treated my older teenage children as adults in training, in much the same way as an experienced mentor teaches skills to young apprentices.*

It has taken us many generations to achieve the society we currently enjoy, but it'll only take one generation to destroy it. We all have a responsibility for the future.

> *Note: Gender equality training starts from the day we're born. There are no gender specific roles, tasks, or jobs. Childbirth is a biological function not a gender task.*

Learning about the different types of personalities will help you to better decide who you are.

Essentially, there are twenty-four distinct personality types. Twelve are female and twelve are male. These personality types are well documented, and I suggest you do some research into this area of study as it is both fascinating, and insightful.

What I've realised throughout my studies, that isn't well documented, is that we as individuals will get along brilliantly with only two of these personality types. One female and one male. This equates to approximately eight percent of the population. We'll get along quite well with a further seventeen percent of the population. So, I'm claiming that we'll get along well with only one in four people. They will be the sort of people that you will want to spend your time with.

The next fifty percent are neutrals. Your interaction with them will be beneficial for the duration that it is occurring, and it'll conclude as soon as it is finished.

The next seventeen percent of people will be automatically disagreeable to you. You won't get along very well, and you may feel uncomfortable in your dealings with them. You may not be aware or understand why this is happening. Their behaviour will be somewhat unpalatable or disagreeable, possibly without you being able to verbalize why. Your participation with them will only occur through necessity, but you will not be comfortable doing so and you will move on as soon as practical.

The remaining eight percent will be totally disagreeable to you, and you will avoid them as a survival instinct. You will be able to understand what it is about them that you don't like. In some situations, you will be tempted to tell others what it is about this person that you don't like. Here, I recommend caution.

The catch, yes there is one, is that you'll need to meet, interact, interpret, evaluate, and decide which people are in what category, and you may not have much time to do this. Inexperience will show, and as you are developing skills you may sometimes end up being with people who you think are friends, but in reality, they are bad for you. Gaining wisdom and experience through having many social interactions, should improve your skill set in working out who is good for you to be with. However, sadly there is a second catch. We are habit forming. We like to be predictable. After three social contacts, even with a person that is totally incompatible to us, will start a friendship trend that will be hard to stop.

This is especially true when forming a permanent relationship that may lead to marriage. Inexperienced people are too quick to form commitments with the wrong type of person and they'll suffer for it. Hopefully, they get themselves out of the relationship before it becomes too difficult to separate.

Even older, experienced people, can fall into the trap by believing that "they know what they are doing." They too can associate with and form permanent relationships with the wrong type of people for them. This is a difficult path to navigate and the reason why relationship breakups are so numerous.

Fortunately, the divorce rate is falling. This could be due to the higher level of public domain advice on relationship problem solving. It could also be that we're less impulsive and take greater care before committing to a permanent relationship than we were in previous generations. It may also be in part that the children who grew up with divorced parents are now more resolved to not let this situation happen to them.

True friendships are invaluable. They create a community of interest in everything.

A big trap that many people fall into, in forming new friendships, is to do so because they believe they can materially gain, or socially improve, by being associated with that person. Don't offer friendship, when you are actually offering a business relationship for mutual gain. Fake friendships are undignified and rob them of all their value.

All your family members can be placed into these twelve female and male personality types. The problem comes when they fall into the categories that clash with yours. Your only course of action is to limit your contact time with them.

> *Quote - "Don't walk behind me; I may not lead. Don't walk in front of me; I may not follow. Just walk beside me and be my friend." Albert Camus.*

~ 5 ~

OUR NEED TO BE IN A COMMITTED RELATIONSHIP.

> *Quote - Understand that happiness is not based on possessions, power, or prestige, but on relationships with people you love and respect. - H Jackson Brown Jr*

For the most part we live in communities. These range in size from hamlets or villages to metropolises.

As tribal sizes grew, humans separated and spread out across the land to balance out our demands we placed on the natural resources. This initially included water, food sources and shelter. Later it included access to quality soil to grow edible foods, raise and manage livestock, and have access to building materials to make shelters.

From the very beginning, individuals found that this was difficult to do on their own. They teamed up with others and worked together. It didn't take long for teams or tribes to be formed, and they worked together to decide where to live, what to focus their time on, and who to accept, or reject from their group. Naturally, as we're not born with equal height, weight, strength, or intelligence, a hierarchy developed, and leaders were either chosen or someone took charge. An order of importance was created, and cliques formed. Weaker and less favoured people became disadvantaged and so some left their group to start another group, but most stayed and suffered in subservient roles.

As groups grew, order and rules were established. Punishments were issued for infractions and a crude form of justice was developed. Enlighted leaders tried harder to protect the weaker and vulnerable members of the group. Some tried to educate the less skilled people so that their value to the group improved, and therefore the strength of the whole group grew with it.

Villages became towns, then cities, and then metropolises. Infrastructure improved to transport, feed, educate and care for the young, old, and sick, grew with it. Leaders became politicians and, in many countries, competed via elections for the privilege to lead based on their merits and popularity.

A big part of belonging is the need to share your life's journey with a partner. Essentially, the majority of us get married or participate in some form of committed relationship.

> *Old saying - Men marry women and hope they won't deteriorate. Women marry men and hope that they'll improve.*

This expression about our relationship expectations is both funny and sad. It has been quoted in various forms so many times because it has an element of truth to it, and that it is sad that we should even hope for it to be true. All of us are getting older, as the alternative is dying. All people do deteriorate with age, this is the consequence of being alive. All people gain knowledge and wisdom through learning and experience. So, as we get older and change are inevitable, it is now that the independent variables kick into the conversation.

We can influence these variables! We can increase our knowledge through structured learning.

> *Observation - The most important subject they teach in schools is comprehension. Learning how to understand something, through listening and reading, is the first essential step toward learning everything else.*
>
> *The second most important subject is questioning. Learning how to frame a question to obtain clear answers and allowing the responses to expand our knowledge into further questioning.*
>
> *The third most important subject is researching. Learning how to go about finding the answers needed, from books and data bases, to improve their understanding.*
>
> *The next important skill they should teach is the art of teaching. This skill both benefits the student and validates the level of understanding of the teacher.*
>
> *Educators should focus on these four areas of learning to improve outcomes for students.*

We should actively seek out beneficial experiences, as through them we can improve our outcomes and lifestyle. We can make a difference to our health through healthy choices in our diet, and we can exercise according to what works best for us. We can develop a positive and productive attitude towards living. By improving these three areas we can live longer and happier lives. If your chosen life partner does the same, and you both choose to do this together as a team, then your lives are truly wonderful. The benefits to the individuals, their children and to the broader community are immeasurable.

> *Tip - The ideal relationship outcome is when you are in a committed relationship that shares mutual unconditional love, friendship, and respect.*

Relationship breakdowns are a huge burden and cost, on our society. So, given that many relationships fail, how do we improve the odds?

The answer is unfortunately, very complex. If it were easy, then there would be much fewer relationship breakdowns and divorces.

There are two important evaluative processes that an individual can use to navigate and thereby reduce the risk of relationship failure. The first part determines your compatibility and the second determines the level of attractiveness.

The first place to start is to define your own personality type. Start by asking yourself these questions.

1. Do you like yourself? Are you the person you want to be, or are you currently evolving into becoming that person? We're always changing, but are your changes random, or are they thought out and planned?
2. Do you know who you are, what you like, and where you are going with your life. Do you have a plan?
3. Do you enjoy learning and expanding your knowledge and experiences or do you prefer a sedentary lifestyle.
4. Do you enjoy hugs, or do you prefer less physical contact.
5. Do you know what you dislike and how to avoid it? Have you learned from prior mistakes?
6. Are you bored? Now is the time to find activities that interest you.

7. What are your attitudes towards work, and do you know what your work ethic is? Are you productive? Have you measured yourself against past experiences, peers, and employers' expectations? (self-employed people with poor work ethics tend not to remain self-employed for long).
8. Are you managing your finances responsibly. Do you spend less than you earn, and do you also consider future needs and wants? Or are you living for the moment with little regard for financial commitments?
9. Are you outwardly focused and extroverted, or are you a quiet, reserved, and modest person?
10. Do you tend to be logical in your decision making and thoroughly think things through or are you impulsive and prefer to deal with the consequences when they happen.
11. Are you family orientated? Do you want children in your life? Do you care for family and friends? Or are you aloof, and prefer to be alone, with little interaction with others?
12. Will pets add stress to your life? If they will, then don't have them, and don't enter a relationship where one will be forced onto you.
13. Are you naturally submissive, passive, assertive, aggressive, or dominating. Are you seeking to control your life, or do you prefer to be led? Are you wary of abdicating responsibility for your own happiness, or are you happy to do so?
14. Are you the sort of person that remains loyal, faithful, and committed to a relationship, or do you prefer a free-spirited approach?
15. Are you energetic, enterprising, and thrive on being productive at home, or at work, and the activities you're doing, or are you laid back, seeking the easiest path and are comfortable with others doing things for you?
16. Do you remain in control when faced with adversity, do you seek solutions to problems, or do you crumble and are defeatist?

17. Can you see the details as well as the big picture, or do you easily get overwhelmed?
18. Do you see yourself as a constructive or destructive person?

When you believe know yourself and are comfortably presenting your true self to a potential partner you are fifty percent of the way there.

The next challenge is to find a future partner who has not only done a similar self-evaluation but that they are compatible with the majority of your responses to those questions. I did warn you this was going to be hard.

Secondly... Sorry, yes there is a lot more to this relationship success formula.

This part is all about attraction. Generally, we humans do part two before we do part one. If only we could be so disciplined and wise enough to do the self-evaluation first, then there would definitely be much fewer relationship failures. However, the vast majority of us rely on attraction, and scantily consider compatibility until after the relationship has started.

Hence the problem.
You should make the time to ask yourselves the following questions about our potential permanent partner.

1. Are you attracted to them? This includes both physical and mental qualities.
2. What benefits will you enjoy from the relationship? Are they similar in passions, hobbies, and interests, and will you be enriched by their past experiences? Do you risk looking boring to them, or they are quickly bored with me because of our mismatched lifestyle?

3. Do they prefer travelling and exploring, or are they home bodies?
4. Are they sexy? Do they share a similar sex drive to you? Do they share similar sexual desires and appetites?
5. Are they willing to wait until you know each other better before wanting to be intimate? Or is their interest in you mostly physical? Is sex with them safe?
6. Do they have financial stability? Do they work and earn well? Do they have assets? Are they money wise?
7. Are their plans, goals, personal objectives in sync with your own? Can you discuss this comfortably?
8. Do they want to be parents one day? Find out early as this can be a deal breaker.
9. Are they kind to animals and care about the environment, or are they indifferent?
10. Are they generous, measured, or stingy, with their money?
11. Are they flexible, rational, and reasonable about life activities, or are they controlling and prefer telling instead of discussing.
12. Do they want to be in charge, are they collaborative, competitive, combative, or do they prefer to be submissive?
13. Are they prone to anger and frustration when they don't get their way? How well do they cope with setbacks?
14. Will you lose your identity to them and feel that you only exist in their shadow?
15. Do they have a compatible style of humour, and can they surprise you in pleasant ways? Or is your time spent with them filled with groans and disappointments?
16. Do you have fun being with them? Do they make you laugh? Are you happy in their company?
17. Is silence awkward between you, or can you be happy just being together?
18. Do you like their family and the level of control they have on your potential life partner?

19. Who are their friends and influencers? Do you also like and trust them?
20. Are they calm in a crisis and focus on the solution or remedy, or do they add to the problem.

Phase two questions are very important and a failure in finding sufficient quality and desirable responses to phase two questions should be an immediate deal breaker. Run, don't walk. End it now and find someone more suited to you.

But wait. There are even more questions. This third category may seem harmless enough, but incompatible responses will exacerbate as your relationship progresses, in particular when you reach the stage of cohabitation.

The phase three questions are.

1. What are their habits and routines?
2. Do they have compatible manners?
3. What are their personal hygiene preferences?
4. Are you both comfortable enough to discuss things like farts? You can't hold them in.
5. How critical is their body shape to your desire to be in this relationship? It will change over time.
6. Are you comfortable with how clean their home, car, and cloths are? Do they respect possessions the same way you do?
7. How well do they treat other people that are serving them? Do they do so in a way that works for you?
8. Do they have annoying mannerisms or witticisms?
9. Are they compatible intellectually?
10. Are they capable of offering a sincere apology to you when they are wrong and may have hurt your feeling?

> *Caution - Domestic abuse and Domestic violence is a major relationship problem. Look for the early warning signs that this may feature in your relationship. If they are evident, they'll generally get worse over time. My suggestion is to end the relationship and avoid becoming a victim. It is your responsibility to stay safe and to stay sane. Protect yourself and any children that you already have or may have in the future.*

The final check list is perhaps the most important. Try to do this one before making a permanent relationship commitment.

The five most important aspects of a successful relationship are.

1. Love. True love is unconditional. It is accepting of setbacks, and you'll have a sense that love resides in your soul.
2. Friendship. The type that is trusting, understanding, supportive, and encouraging.
3. Respect. In each other's beliefs, skills, and actions.
4. Trust. In everything you both do.
5. Time. The longer you are together, and the more evidence you have that the other four aspects are real, the more committed you'll become to your relationship.

Do this quick test. Assign a value out of one hundred for how you feel about your partner for Love, Friendship, Respect and Trust. Then do the same for how you feel they value you.

Compare the results. Mutual high scores in each category are preferable. If they reveal a good match, then your fine. If they don't, then it may be time to re-evaluate your plans.

By asking yourself all these questions, and by trusting, and acting on the answers, you will greatly improve your chances of living in a successful relationship.

> *Tip: If you are fortunate to be in the group of people who can report that enjoy life in a wonderful relationship......., don't mess it up.*

Then why aren't more people asking them and trusting their answers? Sadly, the truth is that even if we were thorough and asked ourselves all of these questions, we'd still make bad decisions about partners. It often takes a full year to truly learn another person properly. As I've stated before, we're creatures of habit and are predictable.

Some relationships will deteriorate and may even fail. Sadly, people will suffer.

I can only hope, that by reading and applying what you learn from this book, or other books similar to this one, that you can improve the odds and reduce the risks. I'd like to believe that your families, and the whole community, will thank you for it. At the very least, you'll improve the odds of achieving a happier life.

So why do relationships fail even if we did ask all the right questions and made the appropriate decisions? We're instinctively a rationalising species. We're hopeful that negative attributes about others are only temporary, and that their true self is a better person than what they currently exhibit. We're driven by hormones, and the need for physical intimacy can entrap us into a relationship with very few redeeming qualities.

Strong reasons for not getting into a relationship or becoming married to that person.

1. When it is only for material gain for you or for your children.
2. To improve your social status.
3. Out of fear or retribution. Don't be bullied into marriage.
4. When it is only for the purposes of immigration or preventing deportation.
5. When parents have commanded it.
6. In order to spite your family.
7. To thwart another suitor.
8. When it is only lust driven.
9. When it is only to assuage loneliness.
10. To win a dare or a bet.
11. When it is only to have children.
12. When an unplanned pregnancy guilts you into the permanent relationship.
13. If courtship is dominated with bickering, arguing, or even constant contradicting, especially in front of others, end it now!

> *Tip: Be truly in love with the person you choose to conceive a baby with. Make certain that this feeling is mutual.*

Humans are habit forming. We tend to stick with what we know even when it is detrimental to our physical and mental health and happiness. Some of us fear being alone. We believe a bad relationship is better for us than no relationship at all. We often fear the unknown. New relationships can be scary. Especially if we have been out of circulation for a while. We may end up being in a worse relationship the second time around. Many of us are doomed to making mistakes as we didn't know any better.

We often fear disappointing, or emotionally hurting the other person, as well as fear the possible retribution for doing so (real or imagined).

The number one reason why so many of us end up living in low value relationship is that our catchment area is very small. We don't actually get to meet many people and so we have few to choose from. Our experiences in relationships are often limited. Some of us started our life partner commitments as young adults and we were not even aware of who we are or what values were important to us. We had no idea of knowing the type of person we wanted to be with. Couples who consider themselves to be in great long-term relationships think of themselves as being lucky. By asking ourselves these evaluative questions, we can improve the odds.

> *Privileged advise - At a wedding that I attended, the priest gave the bride and groom some advice that resonated with me. He explained that as a married couple that they were entering a new phase of their lives. The years will quickly pass, and that when they reflect on their lives together, that those memories should include each other being involved in that memory. Being a couple meant doing things together, growing closer, being happy together, doing fun things, solving dilemmas, and enriching their lives by being best friends as well as being a married couple.*

The benefits to both participants being in a happy relationship are enormous.

A switched-on, totally committed couple can achieve more as a team than they can as two individuals. They can have an amazing life together. I describe this as 1 + 1 = 3

A functioning couple sharing resources and cooperating will have a good life together. This can be shown as 1 + 1 = 2

A dysfunctional couple who prefers to think and act independently can be shown as 1,1.

A couple who are at constant odds with each other are shown as 1-1=0. At this level there is only unhappiness. Time to change or move on.

A destructive couple -1-1= -2. Time to move on.

> *Tip: Tell the people you love that you do love them. It is also very beneficial to sometimes tell them why you love them. True love shared can move mountains.*

There are many books written on this topic. Some mean well but do little for the reader. Do your research and find the books that resonate with you as they'll help. Everyone's circumstances are unique, so all individuals' needs are unique also.

Those people that experience a traumatic relationship breakdown will benefit from independent customised professional assistance. The biggest barriers to achieving success when utilising these professionals that apply equally to both of you are –

1. Your mutual agreement that you want help, and that you want a solution to your problems.
2. Remaining calm by being able to leave your negative emotions out of the discussion.
3. Your ability to be truthful about all of the problems and who or what created them.
4. That you can discuss and accept your contribution to the problems.
5. Detailing and dealing with issues and events that the other person might still not be aware of.
6. Knowing what it is that you both want from the solution. Do you share the end goal?
7. Your acceptance, understanding, and compliance with the advice given.

8. Remaining positive and committed to making it work, despite experiencing setbacks. Or
9. Agreeing to disagree and dissolve the relationship with the least amount of emotional and financial damage and repercussions.

~ 6 ~

GIVING AND RECEIVING.

> Quote - Running away with all of your mistakes means you'll forever be in bad company. - Stephan De Jonghe

> Quote - Give people more than they expect, and do so cheerfully - H. Jackson Brown Jr

> Rule: When capitulating, do so graciously. Stephan De Jonghe

I have heard it said many times that relationships are about give and take. I've never been in favour of this concept. It brought about too many inequities and I've struggled with it for a long time. I eventually concluded that the sentiment should be that effective relationships are about giving and receiving.

Firstly, in a give and take scenario, the taker often takes more than is deserved or needed. The giver can feel drained and used. Children brought up in this environment tend to be consumers of other people's efforts without reasonable contribution.

Secondly, the giver may work on the assumption that the giving will be reciprocal. In a commercial transaction this needs to be true, or the contract is invalid. In a relationship this stage of equitable exchange isn't expressed, so it is often abused. There are victims who feel devalued, taken for granted, and they are generally unhappy.

To negate this, parents often offer a reward in exchange for performed chores. With young children the equitable nature of the transaction was deemed unimportant and irrelevant. The parent felt they were teaching responsibilities and values. From the child's perspective however, the rewards were a source of income and booty. They were easy pickings. Many children grew up to become adults with these entitlements and continued to take disproportionate to their contribution with their partners or spouses.

History lesson – Early contract laws came about during the ancient Greek and Roman times who documented the rules of transactions, the remedies for failure, and the process of arbitration and mediation when differences were unreconcilable. Leaders recognised that the domestic principles of give and take in a relationship were very inadequate in business, and so they made laws making the exchange legal, equitable, and enforceable.

Families who participate in giving and receiving tend to be more equitable and therefore happier with the transaction process. Children who are taught that chores are a part of life, and that everyone needs to participate according to their age, capacity, and skills sets, without being paid, or rewarded, will more often develop a better work ethic when they are mature enough to enter the paid workforce.

Relationships where spouses and partners participate in equitable giving and receiving are happier and more relaxed. Equitable relationships reduce stress. Giving, or sharing, is one of the main benefits of being in the permanent relationship. Reciprocating provides the giver respect and dignifies the process.

Receiving gracefully involves gratitude and encourages further giving. The upcycle here is that domestic relationships that care and provide for each other, are happier, and more functional.

~ 7 ~

HOW CONSTRUCTIVE IS YOUR CRITICISM?

> *Quote - Raise your words, not your voice. It is rain that grow flowers, not thunder. - Rumi - 13th Century Persian poet.*

Words have significant power so choose them wisely. Use intelligently, they can subdue opposition without the use of force or cohesion.

The words we choose to utter in our lifetime determine who we are and how others perceive us, and therefore how we are treated. Some of us are better than others in forming ideas into words, but all of them have consequences. Do you think before you speak? Do you consider the consequences of what you are saying and how you are saying it?

> *Observation - Many people say "you shouldn't judge a book by its cover" may be true, but we all do it. When we meet people, we tend to make assessments quickly and only slowly change our opinion.*

> *When meeting a person for the first time we rarely have time to really get to know them properly. We rely on they cue's they give about themselves about how they clothe themselves, what odours they emit, and how well they convey the words they choose to use.*

This is even more true for the words we write, however when writing them out we often have time to consider their consequences before we issue the words and set them in motion. We can edit our writing, but we can't easily edit our talking. This means we're judged harsher on our written words than our spoken words because we had more time to select them in the first place.

A friend once taught me to use spoken words for bad news, and written words for good news.

> *Tip - If you choose to write about a problem or an issue that you intend to send to another person or group, let your words sit for a while. Take time to pause. Come back to them and consider how they'll be received and slowly modify them to make them fit for purpose. There are no backsies in written words.*

There are numerous levels of communication. We need to set our position on the scale below before we open our mouth to talk, as is it more difficult to reset your level once your dialogue has started.

> *Note - The main communication killer is fear of the consequences for either the initiator or responder, or both.*

> *Music quote - Words are like weapons, they can wound sometimes. Cher*

The scale looks like this.

1. Conversation.
2. Suggestion.
3. Observation
4. Discussion.
5. Lecture.
6. Criticism.
7. Disciplinary action.
8. Dismissal.
9. Execution.

Conversation – Essentially, this is talking. I list this one as I feel that a conversation is one that has some purpose, rather than just filling the air with words that have no theme or direction. People often make small talk, to be polite, or for the lack of something purposeful to say. A conversation should have a topic and all participants should want to contribute, and all should perceive some benefit.

We're all guilty of making an issue, or responding to an issue, disproportionately to the actual severity of the problem. It is commonly referred to as making a mountain out of a molehill.

The most common reasons for conversations failing are –

1. Misunderstandings.
2. Miscommunications.
3. Redirection or going off topic.
4. Getting bogged down with semantics.
5. Overuse of Idioms, Metaphors, Irony, Slang, and Sarcasm.

6. Swearing.
7. Raising voice levels.
8. Too much detail.
9. Inattention or distraction.
10. Teasing.
11. Arguing details about irrelevant facts and allowing these to break the flow conversation.
12. Power plays by intentionally taking at a level beyond the known comprehension level of the other person.
13. Feeling threatened or vulnerable.
14. Wounded pride.
15. Having a one-sided conversation.

> Tip: Prior to starting a specific conversation, mutually to agree achieve something beneficial as a result of the exchange.

Suggestion – This is the utterance of a plan or an idea that is offered for consideration. The words "I was thinking..." are often used to preface the utterance so as to not let it sound like a command. The importance here is test the receptiveness of the suggestion and achieve consensus. Encourage participation and refinement. Sadly, this may create a competitive environment and possibly result in the theft of the credit for making the original suggestion. When this happens, it may create resentment. Also, be wary of being that person who devalues other people's suggestions as it discourages their future participation.

Observation – This is when one person shares a thought, or an opinion, with another for the purpose of informing them of something they may not yet know but might need to know. This is not always welcomed, despite it being well intentioned so be selective on what you contribute.

Discussion - The process of talking with another person, or group, for the purpose of exchanging ideas and reaching a decision. This works best when there is an agreed objective.

Lecture – Not to be confused with an educational presentation given to students although I do prefer this method of imparting knowledge and ideas to a group of people. Lecturing in this instance refers a long serious speech especially given as a scolding or reprimand. Often favoured amongst spouses or by parents of miscreant children. Again, be certain of the facts.

> *Personal anecdote – My own two children suffered the torment of the lecture. I felt that they needed to understand the nature of their behaviour by explaining to them why it was wrong, the probable consequences of repeated bad behaviour, the correct way that they needed to behave in the future, and the benefits of following the new course of action. This affectionately became to be known as the "Long Speech". A seemingly terrible fate for a small child, but they very quickly learned to avoid Dad's "Long Speech."*
>
> *As they got older, I was able to accommodate them with a "Short Speech" version, and this was eagerly accepted as the alternative to the "Long Speech." By the time they were teenagers we got it down to a "Consider yourself told." From then on, when dealing with undesirable behaviour, they had the option of Dads "Long Speech," the "Short Speech," or "Consider themselves told." Oddly enough, they always chose the last one.*

Criticism – Is defined as the construction of a judgement about another person's negative qualities. Before you use critical observations, you must be certain of your information. Get the facts and understand them. Determine how the situation came about. Learn who else was involved. You also need to be qualified, or experienced, before your criticism can be respected and have meaning.

Never be critical above your own level of competence, as their counter blow will disable your intent. When being critical of another, especially to a spouse or family member, their response can be very different to your intention. It is therefore very important that your approach to any topic which is important to you, that you deal with it in such a way that the recipient understands the true nature of the discussion.

> *Quote - A person who is unaware they are doing wrong, has no desire to be put right - Seneca.*

> *Sometimes you do need to be abrasive to remove the problem. Just remember that too much rubbing will wear out the recipient. Make your point and move on.*

Disciplinary action – This is when one person deals out punitive actions to teach another a lesson that their words or actions are inappropriate, but that there are still opportunities to rebuild the relationship. This is dependent on the perpetrator accepting their error, acknowledging the disciplinary action, and choosing to make amends. This is at a command level when the issuer has authority over the other.

Dismissal – When you've reached a point where another is no longer a part of one aspect of your life. Separation and Divorce fits into this level.

Execution – Is the level you reach when you no longer seek resolution or restitution. The relationship is over and you're ending it for all aspects of your interactions. Banishment and exile are the outcome.

To deal effectively with conflict you must firstly become at ease with it. It's a bit like playing golf, as frustrating as it might be, you have to relax to do your best.

Some important rules

1. Don't have serious discussions in the bedroom.
2. Don't make critical judgements in the evening. Sleep interruption will exacerbate the problem.
3. Never be critical in front of others, especially children. (This doesn't include a professional, mutually agreed upon mediator).
4. Never use expletives.
5. Never raise your voice.
6. Never strike or threaten violence.

> Quote: Arguments start in conversational tones - Seneca.

~ 8 ~

SELF-DETERMINISM AND WHAT IT CAN DO FOR YOU.

> *Quote: If the grass is greener on the other side of the fence... it is time you fertilised your lawn. - Author unknown. A favoured quote of my wife - Deb De Jonghe*

Firstly, desire what you need and then you can desire what you'd like. Be careful what you strive for as the consequences of achieving the wrong things can be costly, embarrassing, and often irreversible.

Self-determinism is the theory of human motivation, and personality, that states that we are competent to achieve our own personal and collective goals. These include personality goals, wisdom, and material goals. We control our own motivation and with that we can therefore predict our own performance, learning capacity, choose our experiences, and improve our psychological health.

So, how true is it? The short answer is that it is mostly true. During the course of our life there are always going to be setbacks and detractors. When you learn how to make allowances for these, you improve your odds of achieving your goals.

People who take charge of their lives achieve more and are generally happier. A worthy set of achieved goals gives tremendous satisfaction, and personal growth, in both confidence, and wealth.

> *Actions that are unplanned, will produce unplanned results. Plans without actions, are just words.* - Stephan De Jonghe

The meaning of life is to do things. That means we have choices. It starts with thoughts that manifest into ideas. These ideas become plans which develops into goals. This includes where we work, and what type of work we do. Who we form relationships with. Where we live, and in what type of accommodation we choose to live in. What foods and drinks we consume and how much. What clothing we buy, and how much we pay for all of these options in comparison to how much we earn. So be careful what you mostly think about as your thoughts determine where you'll spend the rest of your life and what you'll be doing with it.

The likelihood of success in goal achievement are influenced by the following.

1. The level importance you place on the task. It'll help greatly if you can imagine yourself happily using, or doing, the thing you desire.
2. The more vivid your picture the more likely you'll succeed. Write them down as soon as you think of them. You can edit them or dismiss them latter, but if forgotten they may be lost forever.
3. A goal equally shared with a spouse or life partner has a greater chance of succeeding.
4. The intensity you are prepared to apply to it. Make it feel urgent.

5. The perceived benefit or reward you'll achieve by having it. Give it a duration of how long, or how often, you'll benefit from having it.
6. The consequence of failure, real or imagined. Imagine missing out. Avoid regret.
7. The level of prior knowledge or understanding of what you are seeking.
8. Your desire to learn and do research to add to your perception of understanding.
9. Your ability to learn and apply that knowledge.
10. The external influencers who want to assist you. It'll depend on the level of intensity of their desire to assist you, their capacity to do so, and their skill sets.
11. The external influencers who appear to want to thwart your goal through rules, regulations, or competitiveness. If this is intense then there is higher probability that you'll be stopped for whatever reason, especially if what you desire is illegal.
12. Your ability to be flexible when presented with variables or options.
13. The availability of the object or skill that you desire. If it is not available the result will be null, unless you are prepared to invent it, make it, or create it for yourself.
14. The cost. Is it within your current budget. The more affordable, the easier it is to achieve.
15. Your ability to move around a temporary setback.

This will work on anything from buying a sandwich to buying a multi-million-dollar business. The more you want something to occur, and the greater the focus you place on achieving it, the more likely you'll achieve the desired outcome. Just don't neglect the necessities.

The most important component is that you must visualise owning the item. You must imagine your happiness when using it, or gifting it. The more real you make that feel, the more focused and driven you'll be in obtaining it.

It is important that you take steps to avoid buyer's remorse. This is a feeling of regretting the purchase once made. Often quoted as "Be careful what you wish for, as you might get it." It is more often associated with an expensive item, particularly if there is a long-term financial obligation attached to it. You'll also realise you now have reduced buying power after the commitment is made. Buyers' remorse is exacerbated by friends and family who openly doubt the wisdom of the purchase and claim to know better alternatives. The steps you should take is that you should always do your research, you need to understand the consequences of what you are doing so that you make informed choices.

~ 9 ~

FAITH AND HOW TO USE IT TO YOUR ADVANTAGE.

> *Quote - Faith can move a mountain of changes, but doubt can build an impassable mountain range. - Stephan De Jonghe.*

Faith is defined as having complete trust and confidence in someone or something without factual evidence or proof. Yes, we should now turn around and walk away, perhaps even run.

However, I am disinclined to do that, as when managed correctly, faith can be a very powerful tool that can shape your life the way you want it to be. Remember, faith is asking you to believe without factual evidence or proof.

There are four types of faith to consider.

1. Faith in yourself. This includes learning, exploring and inventing.
2. Faith in others that you know personally. These include mentors, family, and close friends and they come through for you when needed.

3. Faith in a person that you don't know personally such as a role model.
4. Faith in an entity that you can't validate in any other way other than through faith.

Why do I include this in my book? I have several reasons.

Faith is often used to explain our behaviour, but we do so without defining what type of faith we are using.

Faith is misunderstood and therefore requires clarity so we can use it to our advantage.

Faith energises us to continue, despite setbacks.

Faith inspires others.

Faith in yourself.

This is when we had no evidence of success even before we started, but we did so anyway.

1. Consider explorers. They left their homes and comforts to seek out new life and other worlds. They had little or no evidence before they departed, but they had faith and for many, it paid off.
2. Consider migrants. With little or no evidence, they relocated themselves, and often their families, to start a new life in a strange country and many prospered as a result.
3. Consider inventors. All of them had faith in an idea. Even the successful ones had numerous failures, and each learned from the mistakes, but eventually their faith paid off.
4. Medical researchers who had to have faith in finding the cure. Many didn't know what the journey would look like when they started, and most were surprised by the answer.
5. Chemistry was learned by experimentation. Faith in finding a usable and beneficial outcome was their goal.

6. Starting a business requires an initial leap of faith. Certainly, you can mitigate risk through knowledge, research, financial preparedness, and passion.
7. A student starts a learning program having the faith that it will be completed, remain interesting, be beneficial, and that they'll achieve meaningful and rewarding employment as a result of doing it.
8. Starting a new job, particularly one that is in a different field to your previous experiences, often requires a leap of faith.
9. An author writes and gets books published having faith that they'll become popular with readers.
10. Politicians enter politics with the faith that they can make a positive contribution.
11. Campaigners embark on a course of actions to bring about change, doing activities to increase awareness and improve conditions for those that they are campaigning for even when they aren't personally aggrieved.

The list is endless, and in each example, all of them required having faith in the individual. Most initially fail, but with faith, and persistence, they continue to learn, and history records details of those that prevail.

When having faith in yourself and applying that faith properly to your life, and to your goal achievements, it can be the difference in making the seemingly impossible, possible.

Faith in others that you know personally.
We may not have evidence based on prior outcomes, but it makes it easier to have faith in them if you do.

1. Faith in a family member or members to come through for you when you find yourself lost emotionally, or financially.

2. Believing that the person who hired you will be a good boss, and that you'll like the job and the organisation that employed you.
3. Believing that the person you just employed will be a good fit for your organisation.
4. When you read the synopsis of the book you are now holding, you had faith that I, as the author, had something meaningful to write, and that you'd gain benefit from it. You're still reading, so that's good.
5. Having faith in a person to become your future mentor.
6. Teachers.
7. Medical and health providers.
8. Priests and their equivalent, according to your religion, at the venue you attend.
9. Tradespeople and other service providers.
10. Having faith in a new relationship and for that person to become a close friend or even a spouse.
11. Having faith in a future business partner.
12. I even consider marriage a leap of faith.
13. Buying a house is also a leap of faith.

Again, this list is endless. We rely on our faith that these people will come through for us. Sadly, they may let us down. Before the journey started, we can reduce risk through research, formal agreements, and legal contracts, but the initial decision was based on having faith.

Faith in a person that you don't know personally.
We may have faith in them purely because of who they are. We follow their example, and they are role models to many people. This is despite the fact that we don't know them personally and they don't know we exist. Examples are…

1. The Monarchy.
2. Movie and TV show personalities.
3. Musician's and other entertainers.
4. Sports performers and coaches.
5. Authors, poets, artists. Their works might inspire you, but you need to know them personally to have faith in them.
6. Adventurers'.
7. Specialists in such as motoring, fishing, camping.
8. Politicians and community leaders.
9. Business leaders, inventors.
10. Church leaders.
11. Influencers on social media.

With this group we must restrain ourselves from becoming obsessively interested in them because of who they are, or what they do. They may be interesting, inspiring people, but they are not interested in you because they don't know who you are. Here, any faith in them is probably misguided. It can only change when you do get to know them personally.

Faith in an entity that you can't validate in any other way other than through faith.

> *Observation - This is the part of the book that can land me in trouble, as it may be at odds with the beliefs of this fourth type of person who are faithful to a religion.*

1. Many people have faith in an entity that they have never met, have no recorded evidence that anyone has ever met them, and have no certainty that they ever will be met.
2. They live lives based on their existence and follow and obey human interpretations of their messages.

3. They often gather in groups to share interpretations of these messages and congratulate each other on their acceptance of them.
4. Some people even venerate their organisations leaders.
5. Many alienate doubters or sceptics.
6. Many people work to support the organisation dedicated to promoting truth about the entity, through personal sacrifice of wealth, time, labour, and free will.
7. There is often competition with rival groups with similar doctrines. Over the course of history this can sometimes become violent.
8. Their ethical and moral position is often at odds with the legal code, and this creates confusion for both followers and non-followers.
9. Some faith-based organisations have taxation advantages, creating more confusion as it appears to non-believers that the government is financially supporting behaviour that is contrary to the laws of the land. Reduced taxation also gives them an unfair competitive market advantage that reduces the ability of other businesses to compete.

Note - The formal name for a religious sceptic is an atheist. These people believe there are no deities and publicly thwart those that do. Problems present when they take actions on this belief in ways which are contrary to theists.

An Agnostic, however, is a person who believes that nothing is actually known about the existence, or the nature of God. They believe that faith is not proof, but they may subscribe to a religion for its other benefits.

> *Note - A Humanist is a person who only subscribes to the belief that scientific observation is their proof and achieve legal, moral, ethical, a high standard of values, to lead a happy, dignified, and productive life, without supernatural influences.*

This final aspect of faith is, and should always remain, an informed personal choice. Hopefully, you'll never be pressured or coerced into following this type of faith against your free will.

More details about religious faith: The Holy Trinity is the standard of Christian Orthodoxy. This means it is generally accepted as doctrine, and therefore actively practiced. If you don't believe in the Holy Trinity, you are considered to be a heretic by religious believers. The Trinity is the Father, Son and the Holy Spirit (or Holy Ghost). The Holy Spirit is God Almighty, the Third Person of the Trinity, and the eternal Creator of all things. Scriptures teach that the Holy Spirit is a divine person, and many Christian philosophers prefer to think of God as an unembodied mind.

Why is religion so popular despite its reliance on having faith in an immaterial being? That's easy. Believing in God gives us hope. Hope for a better deal, a better world, and the hope for a salvation from tyranny. Problems present when individuals adopt "blind faith." Blind faith is **trusting in something without any evidence or understanding**. It has been described as a leap in the dark, a giving over of oneself into something despite not having a solid foundation.

Religious teachings explain that God does not expect us to have blind faith, yet very few people who claim to be religious actually understand the principles behind their chosen religion, and so, they do so blindly. Hence my difficulty with this type of faith.

So many allegedly religious people are willing participants of numerous miss-deeds. They participate in religious discrimination, commit anti-social behaviour, undertake criminal activity, and they even sometimes claim to be doing so in the name of their faith. When they do so, they distort public perception about religion, its benefits, and beliefs.

If all religious people were also good and responsible people, then the benefits of being faithful to this fictitious entity would clearly justify their belief. Caution: if you choose to be disbelieving in other people's faith in their religion, then I do strongly recommend that you do so in a respectful way.

So why is religion still so popular?

1. Some participate out of fear of the unknown. They fear retribution in the afterlife.
2. Many just want to feel that they belong to something worthwhile.
3. Research into the stress levels of regular attendees to church services demonstrate that they suffer less stress and have fewer stress related illnesses and a faster recovery rate from heart surgery to cancer survival. Their faith helped them.
4. Religious institutions do great work managing hospitals, schools, aged care facilities, refuges, rehabilitation centres, and they provide moral and financial support to the needy.
5. Religious services offer hope, guidance, and comfort to those in need, most often without payment or reward.
6. Religion offers moral redemptions from sin. Many sins are actually crimes. Some would like to believe that the religiously redeemed sinner ultimately surrenders themselves to the authorities and takes legal responsibility for their actions.
7. Much of the religious teaching stem from Ancient Philosophy and Mythology. This makes it comforting and credible.

The Serenity Prayer is a vivid example of how ancient wisdom has been adapted into scripture.

"God, grant me the serenity to accept the things I cannot change,
The courage to change the things I can, and
The wisdom to know the difference."

I'm not anti-religious. I do have problems with sinners who hide behind religious faith, and I also have problems with those who have blind faith in something they don't understand.

> *True Story - One*
>
> *As a nine-year-old my parents and I went on a country drive. We were living in the Eastern Highlands of Papua New Guinea. My father was working as an Air Traffic Controller at the Goroka Airport. A Controller based in Mount Hagan in the Western Highlands had a car, a Volkswagen Beetle, in Goroka that needed to be driven to Mount Hagan. My dad offered to do this as a family adventure. In return dad's friend would fly us back to Goroka in his light airplane. The journey was only 178km long. On today's roads, the journey takes about two and a half hours. Our journey took place in 1969. The road was made from rammed earth and there was very heavy rainfall. On a very steep and winding section of the road, just near the Chimbu River, heavy haulage trucks became bogged in the mud in front of us and behind us. We were stranded. The floor of the car was rusted, and mud was now seeping through the floor. The mud under our car started sliding down the slope, and some men came and helped us and pushed our car onto level ground. I don't remember how long the journey took, but I do remember that I was very scared. I vividly remember that I prayed, and that I had a strong feeling that my prayers were being answered. Our time in Mount Hagen was fun, and the flight home to Goroka was an amazing experience that I'll always treasure.*

True Story – Two

My career has had its fair share of highs and lows. True to myself, and my resilience, I have always, (so far) bounced back, wiser for the experience. One particular low point of my work was when I surrendered a secure job for the excitement of a business venture. My partner made cakes. The best cakes imaginable, the type they serve in five-star restaurants. My role was to sell these cakes and to develop the range into supermarket offerings. We were going to be rich. I bought myself a six-year yellow Toyota Corona wagon and the business paid for my fuel. Things started to go bad after a couple of weeks. My partner had no money. Suppliers were badgering us for payment. Over the thirty-nine weeks we were together, twenty-six of my payroll cheques bounced. It affected my young family, our ability to pay our loan repayments and we were in financial stress. The business partnership was a big mistake.

It took some time, but I eventually moved on and I ended up in a low status, permanent job, with a very average income and a company car. My career peak was behind me, and I was only thirty-five years old. I was angry at the world and the mess I had made with my career.

Returning home from a business trip to Albany, I drove north on the Albany Highway, daring God to prove to me why I should be happy. Just at that point, my old yellow Toyota Corona wagon, driven by the two ladies that bought the car from me, passed me heading toward Albany.

I looked up and said, "Thanks God, I got it in one."

~ 10 ~

FATE AND WHY WE NEED TO UNDERSTAND THE CONCEPT.

> *Quote - Fate decides who comes into your life: your heart decides who stays. Author Unknown*

Fate is the belief that all events that take place in our lives are predetermined as if by some supernatural power. A Fatalist is a person that believes that this is true and lives their life by it. They consider cancer as inevitable or that people will have accidents or will be wrongly accused. They tend to be less involved in improving the human condition because they feel powerless to intervene and make a difference. It stems from the knowledge that life is fatal. It ends in death and therefore life itself is inconsequential.

Fatalists were once very popular, but this was before science gave us a better understanding which increased our options.

Few people are born with their destiny pre-planned. Those few that are, are most likely miserable.

Yet, old habits die hard, and many of us still linger with some belief that fate plays a part in our lives. In this part of the book, I'll share my reasoning why this remains true for many people, but I want to stress here that it isn't true at all.

If you're not interested in fate, you can skip this negativity and move on to the next part of the book.

> *Observation: When I'm running late to get somewhere, I seem to get an endless stream of red lights and traffic congestion. If I leave early, it's green lights and easy driving. Even though it is only a coincidence, it feels like fate is trying to teach me to be better organised.*

Okay, so you're still reading and learning. Good for you.

The level of fate that we believe in comes directly from our childhood. The more controlled we were in our formative years, the more likely we are, that we'll believe in having a fate, or a pre-destiny. As an infant our every move was controlled by someone else. They decided everything for us as we had no capacity to feed, wash or clothe ourselves. If they wanted to feed us too much salt and sugar, we ate it uncomplaining. If they wanted to dress us up in clothing, however impractical, but for their amusement, then we went along with it. They took us to where they wanted us to be, and they decided who would care for us in their absence. From the moment we were conceived, our fate was being determined by them.

As we grew older, others determined where we would learn and what we'd be taught. Undesirable behaviour and qualities were being measured by adults who often didn't have the skill sets, or experiences, to do so expertly and with confidence. Many parents are guessing what values, behaviours, and qualities to invoke on their children. As children, we don't know any different, and so we accept them all as part of our fate.

Later, we begin to compare ourselves to others. We perform gap assessments. We look at our lives and determine if we are better off, or worse off than others. We begin to question why.

It is at this stage that parents will either brag about how they are better than other parents or resent that they are seen as worse than other parents. Be mindful here as it is only a comparison to the others that are within the periphery. It is not a comparison against optimal behaviour, or nurturing, which is often hampered by a shortfall in desire, resources, and skills.

Shortfalls often inspire resentment, bitterness, apathy and breeds lower expectations. It is at this point that the individual accepts that their current circumstance is their fate or destiny. We rationalise that my parents were like this, so I am too. My parents voted this way, so I do too. My parents follow this team, so I do too. Often, any individual deviation was at best frowned upon, admonished, or at worst banned.

The belief and acceptance that much of our lives are fated comes from how we were treated as a child.

Well-developed children were taught options, and optimal decision making, from a very young age. Their self-determinism was guided so they could learn right from wrong, disseminate the variables, and they knew they had choices and how to make the right ones for them.

Improving those choices, and outcomes, is what the meaning of your life is all about.

Quote "Self-esteem is about you." – Stephan De Jonghe

~ 11 ~

OUR NEED FOR AFFIRMATION.

> *Quote - Humans are too busy rationalising to be rational. - Stephan De Jonghe*

Definition – Affirmations are positive statements that are used to boost our confidence, self-awareness and motivation.

> *Caution - False or forced affirmations will make you feel worse. You must want them and believe in them for your affirmations to become reality.*

Our need for affirmation also stems from our childhood. As children we were either praised, ignored, or criticised, by our parents, guardians, teachers, siblings and peers. As we are instinctively trying to please, we learn it is important to conform or exceed others' expectations. We need feedback to confirm that our actions and beliefs conform with our betters' expectations, so we seek out their approval and praise. It is at this point where some of us strive to achieve greater praise by excelling in tasks, academic performance, athletic superiority, and leadership. Our goal was to become the person giving the praise and not being dependent on others to receive it. Praise became more often linked with reward. We were taught the benefits of higher achievement through the rewards ranging from verbal commendations, certificates, ribbons, medals, academic records, cash, material goods, promotion, fame and increased popularity.

At some point during growth and development, some people decided that they should take credit for the good things, or positive outcomes, for things that they didn't do. They would lie or cheat others out of their deserved praise or reward. They would shortcut the process to either achieve their goals faster, or to avoid retribution for their own failings or inactivity's. This is called cheating and the behaviour is discouraged.

> *Side note - In his book - Humankind: A hopeful History, Rutger Bregman demonstrates through extensive research that humans are instinctively kind people. He promotes the notion that humans are essentially decent, and he concludes that as much as ninety percent of people would prefer to do the right thing under normal circumstances. I recommend this book.*

It is very important that you never abdicate responsibility for your own happiness onto another person. Many spouses and permanent partners find themselves in this situation. Habits are formed and because most people don't like change, the dominant relationship persists. Once surrendered, control over your life and happiness is very difficult to regain. It is your life, so make it your mission to be happy living it.

> *Tip - Make your future goals ones that expand on your current goals. - Stephan DeJonghe*

Ask yourself these questions. Do you like yourself? If you meet you as a person, would you want to be friends? If you project self-distain, don't be surprised when others share that opinion.

> *The only status value judgements that count, are the ones you give yourself.* -Stephan De Jonghe

~ 12 ~

WHY THE WORLD SEEMS TO BE A WORSE PLACE TO LIVE IN THAN IT ACTUALLY IS.

> *Quote - Make ignorance your daily opponent, indifference your constant foe, and prejudice your lifetime enemy. - Author unknown*

The good news is that this isn't true. The world is actually a wonderful place to live. We have everything we need, and all humans can live fulfilled lives with their families and friends if they are left alone to utilize their available resources. When a resource is in short supply, humans find a way to trade for it by either an exchange of goods, or the provision of labour, in exchange for those goods. The use of currency helps measure the equitable nature of these transactions.

It became more difficult when people decided to work out boundaries for which they controlled. The equitable spread and access to resources became impinged. Permissions became required to cross the boundary and some reason or benefit was required to enable a peaceful transaction. Leaders decided to protect this boundary and to protect the resources and the people under their control.

> *Opinion – The environment is changing, but not for the better. All life is at risk from these changes. As we become more reliant on Artificial Intelligence, a common concern is that sometime in the future, A I will conclude that humans are the problem, and plot get rid of us. Shouldn't we focus on using artificial intelligence to benefit all lives, including plants and animals. Shouldn't we alter the narrative to benefit all of us and not control our future?*

So why do we feel less confident about the future. Pessimistic attitudes are more prevalent and so is diagnosed depression. We are in a mental health crisis. Why is this happening when we have an abundance of all of life's needs.

The first problem is the distribution of wealth. A minority of people are enjoying an excess of everything. Too many people have little or nothing. The haves are too scared to accept their part in the problem and will not willingly reduce their excesses. Only rule of law prevents a revolution.

The second problem is scaremongering. Our politicians, leaders and the media, constantly reinforce the messages of global threat, strife, unrest, protest, crime, disaster, disharmony, to a point where we receive more bad news than we do good news. These constant repetitions of the problems facing humanity alter us permanently into a state of paranoia. Good news represents a minority of our news coverage, but in reality, good events occupy more than ninety percent of human activities.

> *Observation - There are many regions across the world where the inhabitants are doing it tough. The vast majority of the global community want to help, or at least want help and better outcomes for those people. Our government leaders often focus on sovereignty when collectively they should be focusing on improving the human condition. We need to improve the average happiness, health and opportunities for everyone. History teaches us that global trade unites and improves outcomes. War divides us and through the premature death and destruction there are many losers. Sadly, when evil prevails, good people, despite being in the majority, hide.*

Why are human's bad news magnets? Why is it true that bad news sells newspapers. Why are we fascinated with events distant and remote to our own lives that are bad for other people? The answer to this is that we are fascinated with what might happen to us one day. We examine the plight of others so we can prepare to avoid it. We secretly take some solace in the fact that we are not part of the tragedy. "Oh, look at those poor people, I'm glad it isn't me or a loved one."

The solution is sadly simple. Wealthy people need to lower their expectations. We need an improvement in the distribution of wealth. We need a benevolent regime that is focused on society's needs, and not focused on wealth creation, and we need to properly and positively communicate this to everyone. The benefits would be enormous and quickly dispersed. It doesn't take much to improve a person's life.

History, however, teaches us that this is just a foolish idealistic dream and that it won't happen. It should, but it won't. Even as an optimist I know this to be true.

> Quote – *If history teaches us anything it is that nobody learns the lessons that history teaches us.* – Robert A Heinlein

The important consideration is that you should constantly take steps to improve your happiness, success in goal achievement by refining your plans and mitigating setbacks. Many spouses discover their true capacity for success only after their marriage is over. Many people wait to be kicked out of a bad job before embarking on a more productive and rewarding enterprise or career in their new job.

Don't wait for a bad experience to make a positive change.

We buy insurance before we need it, in the hope that we don't. Start improving your knowledge and skills now while you can, and don't wait until you have too. Spend time, thought, and energy on yourself. It's your life and your responsibility.

If you can achieve this with a life partner, then that's even better.

~ 13 ~

SIX EMOTIONS YOU SHOULD LEARN TO MINIMISE.

Greed or Avarice. This is when you have an uncontrollable longing for an increase in power over others, or an increased ownership of material things. It creates undesirable conflict and anti-social behaviour. Greedy people are disliked, alienated and often thwarted.

Jealousy. This is a condition when you feel miserable because another person is receiving the affection or attention that you feel you deserve. It is brought on through thoughts of insecurity and fear of losing a significant others love and respect. Its use as an emotion is mostly self-defeating, as through its application you'll turn those very people away from you. Jealous people are often pitied, despised, and alienated.

Envy. The emotional pain you feel when you learn of another's good fortune. It can stem from them having a material thing, realizing a significant achievement, or having a superior quality. Outwardly envious people are often despised and alienated.

> Quote – The rich would relax more, if they only considered how burdensome it is to be poor. - Seneca

Hatred. Intense opposition to a thing, or an idea, or a person. The person feels a revulsion and is often angry and disgusted by it, or them. Often, this is a taught behaviour and is characterised by a lack of understanding or extreme ignorance. Experiencing uncontrolled hatred can result in poor decision making that leaves the user worse off for expressing or acting out their intense hatred. People who hate are often too focused on the object of their hatred and miss out on opportunities and beneficial aspects of life. Haters are often out of sync with community values and are alienated.

Anger. An intense response when feeling hurt, threatened, frustrated, or aggressively thwarted. It is sometimes beneficial, as it allows you to break through barriers to being heard.

I caution its overuse and that you'll need to calm down quickly once you have their attention and involvement. If used excessively, it can render you unfunctional, lose you respect, earn you contempt, and trigger a greater risk of heart and blood pressure problems.

> Quote – Anger, carried to excess, brings about madness. - Seneca

Regret. Is a feeling of sadness or disappointment over something that was done or something that has failed to be done. Experiencing to much regret over missed opportunities in relationships, careers, and interests is a heavy burden. Sometimes repentance or an apology doesn't cut it. Minimise regret by thinking through the consequences of not saying or doing the thing that your instincts and judgement tells you to do. Once experienced, you best option is to learn from the mistake to improve future decision making.

> Quote: *If only. Those must be the saddest words in the world.*
> Mercedes Lackey - Author

Overcoming, or at least reducing these six emotions is very difficult, particularly if you've had them for a long time and they are a feature of your personality. If you do regularly experience them, and want to mitigate their impact on your happiness, start by learning to reduce the intensity of the feelings you experience when feeling them.

There are specialised books that you can study to help you overcome these emotional disabilities and there are also numerous resource centres, and specialists, that you can turn to, to get professional help.

~ 14 ~

ACUTE STRESS RESPONSES AND HYPERAROUSAL. WHAT DOES IT ACTUALLY MEAN?

> *Tip – Remember to breathe.*

In this part of the book, I'll examine behaviour when a situation or an event occurs, that is physically or mentally, (or both) that is terrifying to us. The purpose of writing about it here, is to fill a gap in the knowledge that I feel exists in the minds of many people.

Acute stress response is your physiological reaction to something that is terrifying to you.

These "Fight or flight," responses to situations are well documented, and they demonstrate how you will react when you are faced with imminent physical danger. You choose between defending yourself or running away. Engage or evade. The decision is triggered by hormones, and it is our evolved way of ensuing survival.

1. The mind is on high alert, and you'll feel agitated and have a sense of impending doom.

2. You'll experience rapid breathing which could lead to hyperventilation.
3. You'll focus on the threat and become oblivious to extraneous activities.
4. Your heart rate will go up and your chest will tighten. You may feel you can't breathe.
5. You'll perspire more and may feel the urge to urinate or defecate.
6. Your muscles will tighten, and you may ball your fists.
7. Blood will drain from your skin, and you may feel clammy.

There is a third response. I call it fright but it is also known as freezing behaviour. The body freezes in fear and simply allows the threat to act out its intention. An example of this is the fear an animal feels when in the spotlight of an oncoming vehicle in the dark of the night. Fear incapacitates the animal, and it gets run over.

Also, there are phobias. This is when there are no threats, but we have a fight, flight or fright response. The perceived threat is sufficient to suffer the symptoms. When faced with a future task that we believe will put us in danger we manifest the symptoms and avoid the situation. An example of this is when a soldier experiences anxiety prior to military action.

There are self-manifested fight, flight, or fright responses. The imagination is a powerful thing. We have the ability to conjure numerous threats and have very real responses to them. Have you ever woken up from a nightmare. The symptoms are the same and if left untreated it can lead to hyperarousal. Studies have shown that up to twenty percent of us have difficulty returning to our normal state after experiencing acute stress.

Hyperarousal is defined as being in a state of increased psychological and physiological tension. It leads to prolonged anxiety, insomnia, accentuation of your personality traits. This is a bad condition, and it needs to be professionally treated. Also known as post-traumatic stress disorder or PTSD.

Threats to your person can seriously impact on the quality of your life and may even permanently affect you. The benefits of understanding this is so that you can mitigate them and perhaps choose to master them.

The decision to fight, flight, or fright, is an emotional one, so therefore by mastering your emotional response under these circumstances, you will reduce the severity and duration of mental harm. You can achieve this by mitigation, preparation, education, and prevention.

Mitigation. Knowing what to do after dealing with a threat and the danger has passed, will impact on the extent and duration of the psychological damage. Deep breathing, walking, talking through the experience with a carefully chosen close friend or mental health professional, meditation, listening to your favourite music, hugs from a loved one, time spent with a pet, working on a hobby, are all good things to do. Avoid medication, alcohol, isolation, and do not participate in self-harm.

Preparation. Our parents started this training when we were very small. Being taught how to cross the road is a great example of how we become prepared to potential threats. Car verses body and the body loses. Being taught potential dangers within the household prepares us for independent living. These lessons can be used to prepare us against all manner of future threats. We can also undertake self-defence courses; we can exercise to improve flight options, and we can give consideration to how we'd respond in various scenarios so that we know what to do. Stoic philosopher's advocate the mental preparation of your planned responses to rapidly unfolding events.

Education, our parents, family members, friends, mentors, and emergency service providers are all willing to teach you the dangers that you need to learn to avoid. You are at most risk in an unfamiliar environment. Risks range from abduction, theft, fraud, all the way to animal attack risks, poisonous plant risk, disease, and injury through misadventure.

Prevention. By researching we can learn threat assessments made by other people who have experienced threats in parks, regions or countries that you may be planning to visit. Agencies and travellers regularly publish warning of the potential dangers.

> *Quote - An ounce of prevention is worth a pound of cure - Benjamin Franklin.*

We can plan for these and prepare for what we'll do if there is a negative event and mitigate the damage thereby improving the quality of the experience and be happier for participating.

~ 15 ~

LET'S TAKE A LOOK AT HIGH ACHIEVERS.

> *Quote - Learn from other people's mistakes as you don't have time to make them all yourself. – Stephan De Jonghe*

> *Quote - The Highway to success is always under construction. Author unknown.*

Some people have turned their responses to hyperarousal into a skill. They have adopted preparation and prevention into an advantage so that they can do an increasing range of activities without experiencing the disability of fight, flight or fright. These can-do people achieve amazing things in their lives, and we can benefit from understanding their approach to life and their ability to achieve so much more than the average person.

> *Quote - Luck is when opportunity meets preparedness. Seneca*

Random luck is rare.

People who have mastered their responses to hyperarousal are also prepared to take advantage of every opportunity that appeals to them.

Often it is through this preparation that you "Make your own luck." By preparing, you meet like-minded people, seek out mentors, and gains skills and knowledge manifesting in confidence to stretch your growth horizons. You may take risks, but you don't leave it to chance. Success comes from applying your preparation to the opportunity.

The main qualities that high achievers have in common are that they are...

1. Positive thinkers.
2. They are organised and have daily routines.
3. Love learning and doing their research.
4. They are driven and highly self-motivated.
5. They use visualisation to imagine the successful outcome.
6. They are highly intuitive and trust their instincts.
7. They act on their plans without hesitation.
8. They establish a new set of goals before the completion of the current goal.
9. They hold themselves accountable for the results.
10. They are vigilant for the opportunity.
11. All of them know what they like doing, and know what makes them happy,
12. They capitalise on what they are naturally good at doing.
13. They are confident and like themselves.
14. They all see setbacks as temporary and when they do happen, they are adaptive and immediately plan for the work around.
15. They walk away from negative environments and negative people.

16. They declutter their mind. The less things they focus on, the clearer the picture.
17. They stay on topic and are focused on relevant answers and practical solutions. They ask a lot of questions, and they really want to understand the responses.
18. They work hard and contribute what they are good at.
19. They recruit the best people who are needed to accomplish their multiple goals.
20. They plan beyond achievement.
21. They are grateful to learn from other people's experiences and from other people's mistakes.
22. Happy to teach others and develop mutually rewarding relationships.
23. Interestingly, all of them believed in the outcome before it happened, and they all thought that they could've done more.

Another common trait amongst truly successful people is that it takes nine to eleven years of commitment, study, and hard work, for them to achieve greatness within their specialised field. The earlier in life that you start this process, the younger you'll be when you reap the benefits.

> *Quote: No one can lead a happy life without the pursuit of wisdom.*
> *- Seneca*

If you can learn to prepare for the unexpected, you'll be better equipped to deal with what comes your way. An example of Seneca's is when you are traveling at high speed, and you see the potential for a pedestrian to cross your path, that you are mentally prepared for what to do if they misjudge their steps, and you can take quicker action to avoid, or at least mitigate collision.

So, there you have it, all written out for you. Your path to greater success and increased personal goal achievement. So why aren't more people doing this?

Sadly, the explanation is very simple. It is much easier to manage our expectations to our current reality, than to change our reality to meet our expectations.

All people are drawn into habits, routines, and comfort zones. It isn't that we are lazy, complacent, or distrusting in the process of change. It is because we haven't sold ourselves on the benefits of exceeding beyond our current situation. All personal growth and change must be desired at a much higher level than our current circumstances. It must be sought after with passion so that we can burst out of the gravitational like field that binds us to our current lifestyle, much in the same way an astronaut's rocket requires enormous energy to escape Earth's gravity. This gravitational like field is so strong, and the mental energy required to break free from its hold, is beyond the desire of many people.

> *Tip - No one likes temporary setbacks, but if you learn how to manage them, you'll recover sooner. - Stephan De Jonghe*

~ 16 ~

WHERE ARE YOU EMOTIONALLY?

> *Quote: Your reputation is more important than your name.*
> Stephan De Jonghe

Emotions are defined as a combination of strong feelings that resulted from your circumstances, your mood, and your relationship with others.

This is important as happy, positive people, tend to be more productive and successful, than sad, negative people. The difficulty is, how do you measure this. Many people can appear happy when they are truly sad. Others may appear cynical but may actually be self-fulfilled and productive. How we see ourselves can be very different from how others see us, or how we allow others to see us.

Anyone who has investigated this aspect about themselves, will tell you that you'll generally feel worse off by knowing. Ignorance can be bliss. Knowing the truth about how others see you can only be beneficial when you suspect you have a problem and are ready to improve. Your own analysis of yourself maybe insufficient in determining who you are, and what you need to do to improve.

Most people will choose to avoid the humiliations that come with this process, and therefore continue to stumble on as before.

We think we know ourselves intimately. We spend one hundred percent of our lives within our own minds and whilst we know we can deceive others, in truth, we shouldn't believe we can deceive ourselves. We think we know our emotional limitations and most of us seem willingly to surrender ourselves to the consequences. We'd like to be a better person. We try to convey behaviour of being a better person to others that we interact with, in particular to those people whose opinion of us has value.

In reality, most of us are living a lie. We're conveying a representation of a person we'd like to be, which can be very different from the person we believe we are. We do this because we perceive that when we are judged as being successful, that the rewards will exceed the risk. Humans are only too willing to gamble with their emotions.

You need to live with another person for at least one year to truly know them. That is how good we are at masking our true selves. One reason for this is that our emotions are in flux. They, like the weather are in constant change, adjusting to the prevailing pressures, desires and disappointments. Emotionally, who you are today may be different from who you are tomorrow, next week or next year.

We analyse this by looking at our average. If you like, you can plot this mathematically. This gives you your own personal emotional score. Keep this to yourself as everyone's individual score is dependent on the day and how much value they place on any particular emotional measurement. We're all different, so how you feel about something, will be different to how other's see and feel about the same thing. We therefore cannot compare our emotional score to others.

We can, however, compare our current emotional score to our own previous emotional scores. The benefit of doing this is so we can plot and plan our personalised emotional improvements.

> *Caution - This can work wonderfully for an individual. In rare cases it can benefit to a like-minded and committed couple, but it can also reveal a plethora of emotions that you didn't know existed about each other. Using it on a group or for a group will end in tears and failure at this point, is essentially guaranteed. Emotional growth for a group takes years and for a society, it takes many generations.*

So, let's look at some examples of your emotions. I've listed them in groups that I regard as positive, neutral, and negative. Your emotional map, or scores, is determined from the way you assign your values to each emotion listed.

This varies from who you are at this moment and who you are with. Whether your outcomes meet, or exceed your expectations, and were your expectations realistic. They are very dependent on how tired you are, what your external stresses are and over what length of time you've had to deal with those stresses. Even what you ate or drank can have a bearing on your current emotional score. It'll also depend greatly on how you were raised and what type of people your parents are and those other people who influenced and shaped who you are emotionally.

Caution - This exercise may seem a little futile as there are too many independent variables for it to be of much value. Please be resilient here. Your emotional map, or score, may reveal things about yourself, to yourself, that you didn't previously realise were there. The more honest you are with your responses, the greater the benefit. Done periodically, a trend will emerge.

When plotting, try as much as possible to determine where you are emotionally at most of the time. Consider your default setting. Where you believe you are most of the time in your head. I'll explain in more detail why this is important after you have mapped or scored your emotions.

> *Note: Acknowledging your own failings is an indicator of good mental health. As a bonus it also gives you a list of what to work on.*

> *Tip – Only by practicing perfection will you become perfect. But first work out if the emotional cost is worth the effort. It may be best to aim for excellent, or very good. Don't aim too low as you risk achieving it, and you'll remain disappointed with how you're living your life.*

To map your emotions, circle the words on the next two pages that best describe how you are under normal circumstances.

Or

You can score them by assigning a value from one to ten above each word according to the intensity you feel when considering the words. When completed this task, add the total for each positive, neutral, and negative word then you can reveal your dominant emotional state.

Positive emotions

Assertive, Affectionate, Joyful, Happy, Jubilant, Delighted,

Pleased, Calm, Confident, Secure, Amused, Tactful, Sensitive

Graceful, Tolerant, Altruistic, Helpful, Reasonable, Loyal,

Productive, Genuineness, Trustworthy, Hopeful,

Energised, Focused, Organised, Balanced, Elated,

Ecstatic, Resilient, Pleased, Proud,

Neutral emotions

Passive, Indifferent, Calm, Nonplussed, Unaffected,

Relaxed, Comfortable, Bored, Dispassionate,

Fair-minded, Inert, Unbiased, Unmoved, Unemotional,

Competent, Indifferent, Disinterested, Unconcerned,

Disinterested, Emotionless, Comfortable, Unresponsiveness,

Negative emotions

Aggressive, Disdain, Morose, Mournful, Sad, Displeased,

Glum, Bitter, Incensed, Bewildered, Confused, Panicked,

Enraged, Angry, Cross, Gauche, Indiscrete, Clumsy,

Judgmental, Greedy, Irrational, Neutral, Treacherous,

Lazy, Cheater, Swindler, Pessimistic, Drained, Distracted,

Jumbled, Unprepared, Biased, Disappointed,

Shattered, Fragile, Jealous, Envious

There are many more emotional words that I could write down, but the above list is sufficient for this exercise. If you circled the words to create your map, or scored the results, you can now see where you are emotionally.

> *Caution - Do not show your results to others or compare your score with others. This exercise is for your benefit only.*

In theory, you shouldn't be surprised by the outcome. The question you now need to ask yourself is, are you happy with the result. Is this the person you want to be. If the answer is yes, then you're fine. You like yourself and you're good to go.

But if your answer is no, and you find that you are lacking positive emotional qualities to be the person you'd prefer to be, then your score becomes your personal foundation for improvement. Research the qualities that you'd like to improve. Get an understanding of what they are, and what they feel like. Seek out people who have those qualities that you admire and try to learn from their example. See yourself as morphing into the person you'd like to be. Do this process very slowly.

> *Caution - Others may notice your personality change. Some will encourage, most will be indifferent, and some will feel confused or even distrusting of it. Slowly change away from your less than desirable qualities and move closer toward those qualities you want for yourself.*

> *Tip - Learn body language. It accounts for at least sixty-five percent of all communication and mastering it will make you a better communicator and help you better understand others. It will help you improve the quality of your life.*

After you have chosen those qualities that you want to change, the process is remarkably easy. Here are a few tried and tested steps toward making the improvements.

1. Start by thinking what those qualities would look like, and how you'd feel by having them. If you don't get excited, and if you don't feel great imagining you're behaving in this new way, then stop now as it won't work.
2. Write them out using those desired qualities in sentences that convey the new reality. Use positive language that describes your elation at having this quality. EG: I'm happy that I convey how pleased I am for others when they describe their achievements, goal completions, or new acquisitions.
3. Look for opportunities to practice this new quality. Don't overdo this or you will appear to lack sincerity and you may be criticised for it.
4. Move on to the next quality that you want to improve and repeat this process until you become the person you want to be.

A temporary setback is when an event, or a person, shifts you away from your normal emotional state. When these events or influences occur, the remedy is to recognise the event, decide that it is temporary, and work toward returning to your normal state.

However, there are a large number of events, that when they occur may have the potential to change your emotional state permanently.

These include, but are not limited to, the following.

1. Forming a deeply romantic attachment to someone and that it is equally reciprocated. (Note - This is often referred to as falling in love. This comes from the suddenness of the onset of this feeling, much like actually falling. The two individuals often feel vulnerable and sense a loss of control through the event. It is therefore exciting and scary at the same time.)
2. The conclusion of a deeply romantic attachment with someone for what-ever reason.
3. Unrequited love.
4. Even an imagined disaster can feel real and cause you to experience genuine symptoms.
5. Death of a spouse, parent, child or close friend.
6. Getting married or becoming separated and divorced.
7. Abandoning a family member due to ongoing unresolvable, and serious issues.
8. Starting a business.
9. Becoming bankrupted.
10. Becoming an addict or dealing with one on a permanent basis.
11. Making a bad career change or becoming redundant.
12. Clinical depression and chronic pain.
13. Living with a chronically depressed or stressed person.
14. Financial windfall or disaster.
15. Permanent illness or permanent disability.

16. Crime as either a victim or perpetrator.
17. Puberty, menopause and midlife crisis.
18. War, natural disaster or revolution.

When these occur, approximately ninety percent of us will be able to recover sufficiently to return to our normal emotional state within twelve to twenty-four months. Sadly, the other ten percent of us will never fully recover. It is impossible to predict how we'll respond emotionally to these events, but hopefully by becoming aware of them, and their impact on your life, you can mitigate the negative consequences. The emotional support of family and friends through this process can be the difference between full recovery and permanent depression, so look-out for each other. We need each other, as we never know when that need will occur.

> *Caution – When enlisting help, make sure that the willing person and also capable. If they are as messed up as you are they'll be company but off little or no benefit too you. Misery may love company, but that using that path will push you further down and delay your emotional recovery.*

~ 17 ~

HOW TO REDUCE EMOTIONAL STRESS AND WHY THIS IS A GOOD THING.

> *Quote - It's not how we make mistakes, but how we correct them that defines us. Rachel Wolchin author of "What you missed while blinking."*

Stress is defined as a mental or emotional strain, or tension, resulting from adverse or demanding circumstances. Interestingly, it can be manifested from both real and imagined sources. Stress is our reaction to threats, challenges, physical, and psychological barriers. Stress is relative to the persons individual skills, experiences and psychological profile. Two people will deal with the situation quite differently. One may see it as a challenge and enjoy the success of overcoming the difficulty, whereas another may allow it to develop into a task that overwhelms them.

Stress causes our body to release hormones into the blood stream. They are adrenaline and cortisol.

- Adrenaline is also known as Epinephrine. The body uses it to control functions of the body which includes an increased

heart rate, and breathing, which allows us to move faster when we are under threat or are excited.
- Cortisol is a naturally produced steroid hormone. It is an essential factor in the proper metabolism of starches.

> *Observation – Some people get so used to having excessive quantities of these two hormones in their system that they actually crave them. They crave conflict and so deliberately exacerbate tense situations because they need the rush that the adrenaline and cortisol give them. They may not even know this is happening to them and therefor have no control over there propensity to exacerbate problems.*

Like many things, hormones in moderation are a good thing. We need them to live. However, in excess they become a bad thing. They work against us and will put undue pressures on our body and mind that we cannot cope with. Prolonged stress is linked to heart disease, strokes, blurred vision, tense muscles, headaches, depression, and it even increases your suicide risk. So, reducing stress is a good thing and by doing so you improve the quality and perhaps quantity of your life.

Some people exacerbate their stress by turning towards alcohol, drugs, overeating especially sugary foods, compulsive sex, unnecessary shopping, excessive internet use, smoking, and other things.

If you think you have a serious problem, then you probably do. Seek help. Read more books on the topic and get professional help. Long term stress can be fatal, and it will certainly reduce the quality of your life and it will also negatively impact on family members. They will become stressed by your stress.

Short term stress can be managed by doing more of these stress reducing activities.

1. Start a new exercise regime or sport.
   1. Ease yourself into it.
   2. Establish realistic goals.
   3. Only spend significant sums of money on it after you've established your love and commitment to that activity.
2. Manage your money. Financial burdens are a major source of stress and relationship conflict. Do a budget, change jobs to earn more money so you can meet, or even exceed your needs. Reduce unnecessary spending.
3. Save some of your money. Having backup money is comforting. When you have spare money, you can reward yourself in some way. This gives you something to look forward to, and it is a positive in your life. This is even more true when it is a shared savings goal that you have with your spouse or partner. Achieving the goal should result in a shared reward. By doing so it will encourage you to do this more often.
4. Reduce debt, especially short-term, high interest, debt. The only two things you should borrow money for are -
   A. Things you can profit on. Do your homework on these items. These include a home, a business, shares, and collectables.
   B. Items that are necessary, but you couldn't reasonably pay cash for them, because of their relative cost. These include a car, weddings and funerals. You can take the sting out of this type of debt by adjusting your expectations. Consider your ability to repay the debt and select the type of car, wedding, or funeral, that fits within your repayment budget. Sometimes the path to greater satisfaction, is to simply lower your expectations.
5. Have a holiday. This one is almost self-explanatory as everyone feels good just thinking about having a holiday. Some rules apply.
   A. Don't borrow money for a holiday. If you can't afford it don't go.

B. Study the destination in terms of their laws and customs. Particularly if this destination is new to you.
C. Consider travel insurance, particularly for overseas holidays.
D. Agree with travel companions the nature of your holiday. Is it for exploring the local scene, or for adventure, or shopping, or simply relaxing.
E. Don't spend money on junk items and keep to an expenditure budget. Beware of hawkers and con artists as they will look for opportunities to steal from people who look inexperienced and vulnerable.
F. Be prepared for when you get back home to your normal life. A great holiday can have a sad ending when you don't mentally prepare for your normal domestic routine.

6. Have a life that focusses on family and friends. We're not designed to do it solo. People living in caring family environments, have less stress and live happier lives. People who suffer prolonged unworkable relationships should consider abandoning them. They'll benefit in the long run.
7. Hobbies and interests are psychologically and possibly also physically rewarding. Some rules
   A. Don't let them add stress to other family members.
   B. Don't let them become expensive. They should be affordable. Set a budget.
8. Be the sort of person who enjoys giving. Keep this in proportion to your ability to do so. Don't suffer yourself or your family by doing so. Receive graciously. When someone cares enough to gift you something of themselves then accepting it in the spirit intended, you up-lift the giver. Devaluing the gift devalues the relationship.
9. It is human nature to seek out equitable outcomes. A win-win scenario sets the stage for more mutually rewarding experiences.

10. Being able to forgive transgressions and move on. Dwelling on a bad experience adds unnecessary stress. This is difficult to do if the event falls into the tragic experiences I described previously. By reminding a person of a mistake, error, or transgression, you replay the negative aspects of the pain you suffered. You lose and they'll lose. Forgive them and you forgive yourself. Measure the retribution in proportion to the problems. Too many children grow up in environments where they believe they are unworthy in their parents' esteem. When they become adults, this burden can stay with them through their adult life.
11. Being prepared and organised can help reduce stress. Feeling confident is an obvious stress buster.
12. Learn from your mistakes. Repeating them is stressful and often expensive. Where possible learn from other people's mistakes, as you don't have the time to make them all yourself.
13. Plan a diet that suits your preferred lifestyle. Engage in an exercise routine that suits you. Don't make this competitive. You're doing this for yourself and not just to be better than someone else.
14. Have regular medical and dental check-ups. Prevention is better than cure and if you can catch a life threating condition in its early stages the likely hood of full recovery is higher.
15. Monitor your self-talk. It is the conversation you have in your head. What are you saying to yourself? Is it positive and constructive? Are you advancing your happiness and productivity? Or are you destroying your world in your own mind? Remember that you will become what you think about. Constant negative self-talk can lead to experiencing clinical depression. The path to recovery is as long as the journey into depression, so don't talk yourself, or allow others to talk you into becoming clinically depressed. Get qualified help early.
16. Develop a can-do attitude. Be aware that emotional stress will hold you back and reduce your happiness.

17. Don't rely on hope to see you through your life's challenges. Friedrich Nietzsche argued that hope was evil as it prolonged torment. Hope for the best, but plan for the worst. Never rely on luck to make your own good fortune. Take charge of your life, give it meaning, and do the things that are important to you, now.

~ 18 ~

SIX IMPORTANT QUESTIONS YOU NEED TO ANSWER ABOUT EVERYTHING YOU DO.

The six questions are Who? What? Where? When? Why? and How? Interestingly, they are all difficult to be properly answered using a "yes" or a "no" response. Journalists, crime investigators, therapists, teachers, and story tellers, love these questions, and use them as part of their mantra. When used properly, they solicit the most usable responses to an investigation, and produce a more thorough and complete understanding of the events.

Where? When? and Who? are reasonably straight forward. When properly corroborated they become factual.

What? is subjective to the perspective of the parties involved and all of the witnesses. Here an investigator needs to triangulate the accounts to gain a clear presentation of what happened. They need to look at what is corroborated and dismiss the improbable contradictory accounts. They also need to take bias into account.

How? is the next question that is subject to examination. Often, there are a series of events that need to be understood as to how the parties involved came to converge, and that needs to be understood.

Why? Why were the people motivated do the things they did leading up to the event. This important question also explains the degree of culpability in an investigation. What were the contributing factors, and can they prove the event as being a simple Misadventure, a Summary Offence, or an Indictable Criminal offence.

Scepticism – Expressing doubt as to the truth of something. Without it the world would still be believed to be flat. It can stem from a conversation, announcement or from written material that you doubt is credible. Scepticism can be both helpful and hurtful so it must be applied with care.

The most beneficial form of scepticism is when it is applied to science and medicine. Topics that are science-based deal in absolutes and the findings need to be examined to such a point where no doubt remains.

Scepticism when applied to an investigation in a criminal matter is that the conclusion is beyond reasonable doubt. An investigator or detective must continue examining the evidence and witnesses, until they are satisfied that a judge and jury would reach the same conclusion when presented with all the details.

Professional scepticism is a skill required by auditors. They need to have an enquiring mind to be able to make critical assessments and consider the sufficiency of the truth portrayed by the investigated.

When you ask yourself these six questions you are actually encouraging yourself to think meaningfully about the responses. Life is rarely about straightforward responses. Certainly, many are, like "Do you want a cuppa"? Many questions and decisions require thought, and by asking yourself these six simple questions you should cover most of the independent variables to achieve the optimum result. The more detail you provide yourself, the clearer the picture, the less likelihood of disappointment.

Couples should perform this questioning together to improve consensus and reduce disappointments. So should management teams. The benefits from asking yourself these six key questions, and remaining sceptical until convinced, should never be underestimated.

> *Tip - Don't let this process become a procrastination tool. Do the research to obtain the information you require then get active using it. Don't become so overwhelmed by the process that nothing happens.*

~ 19 ~

WHY WE SHOULD UNDERSTAND THE LAW, ETHICS, MORALS, AND VALUES.

These are often referred to, and many adults will claim to understand them, but I fear some do not. They are very important aspects of living a quality life and I'll introduce them now so that you can be stimulated to do further learning.

Law
Law – Is a set of rules that evolved over time, that were created to regulate human behaviour, and that they are enforceable by government institutions. Some describe it as "The Art of Justice." This is appropriate as the interpretation of laws requires formal training. Lawyers and barristers do a lot of reading and having advanced comprehension skills is a requirement.

You require formal qualifications to "practice law." They call it practice because, however qualified, practitioners are still learning. These days laws are more altered, then made, and this makes the interpretation of them all the more difficult. Some laws have start dates, and end dates, so the date of the event needs to be taken into account when prosecuting a breach of the law.

The difficulty with understanding law is apparent due to its complexity. If you have a legal problem, get legal help.

Ethics

Ethics – A set of guiding principles that determines what a person, or a group of people will do, and how they'll behave, when conducting a group activity. These are often documented, taught, and even enforced. They tend to be practical and they are often created to protect people from making mistakes when conducting similar or the same activities.

> *Suggestion - Teach Ethics at home. Have a group discussion about what ethics is and formulate an ethical domestic statement that every family member participates in, and jointly agrees to follow.*

Some ideas for a domestic ethics document for your home are:

1. Clean up or clear away items that you have used and return them to where they belong.
2. Respect each other and each other's personal space.
3. Be kind.
4. Ask, and gain approval, before borrowing another family member's stuff and return them in good order and in a reasonable time.
5. Set the volume control at a level that the device requires for your benefit, and not so that it intrudes on others.
6. Accept responsibility for your actions and behaviour.
7. Look after the wellbeing of family pets.
8. Be honest.
9. Participate in family activities for the fun of it and not the competition.
10. Defend each other during outside conflict. Remain loyal to each other.

11. Never contradict a spouse in front of others unless there is an immediate health or safety risk.
12. Look for, and eliminate health and safety risks.
13. Report damages and misplaced items.
14. Do not be envious of other people's skills or their acquisitions.
15. Adopt a balanced approach to helping each other. Don't be a user.
16. Agree to look for solutions instead of only focusing on problems.

> *Suggestion - Ask family members what preferences they have in doing routine chores. Treat them like "want to do's" instead of "have to do's". Encourage the belief that we all need to do our share.*

Morals

These take the shape of a person's perspective about what they perceive to be right, and what is wrong, about anything and everything, and to what degree. Your sense of morality more often stems from your childhood upbringing.

They are self-regulated and subject to constant interpretation. They tend to be an opinion, so one person's morals might be seen to be unacceptable to others. They stem from customs or consistent behaviours that were acceptable at the time in that region. This is where it gets tricky, as morals are the foundation of all laws and ethics. Even criminals can have ethics and no morals. An army will have ethics about killing people and destroying property, even though the individual members of that army will find killing to be morally wrong. Governments will have laws against "Unlawful" killings but will employ people to fight, and kill, on its behalf in military engagements that it deems necessary and then justify doing so. Governments are the biggest killers of human life, yet they claim to be morally and ethically justified in doing so. Some

Governments send soldiers to kill citizens in other countries, which is clearly illegal, and contrary to the laws of both countries.

Unfortunately, sometimes the leaders of one country make a presumption of guilt on the citizens of another, and then attack them without evidence. Go figure.

Fortunately, for the day-to-day activities of many humans, ninety percent of us will gravitate toward doing the right thing. We choose to obey the law, act ethically and morally. We may make a mistake, and we may pay a penalty for that mistake, but we choose to live in a society that has values and rules for our conduct.

Values
The principles of your standards of behaviour when using your own judgement of what is important in life.

Understanding which values are important to you will help guide you toward better decision making and will assist you into making choices that please you.

> *Note - The values you convey directly determine the reputation you'll have. They are a direct connection between what actions you will take when your beliefs are challenged.*

> *Bonus! - If you and your life partner/spouse have shared values, then your homelife will be a lot more productive, happier and healthier.*

> *Caution - You can't force a value onto someone. They either have it, or they want to achieve it for themselves.*

> *Note - Most of our values were acquired during our childhood.*

The Core Values List (there may be others)

My recommendation is that you identify only the core values from the list below that are important for you to focus on developing. If you participate in this exercise, do so in private.

> *Caution - If you choose to do this exercise with a spouse/life partner, and then afterward compare your values with theirs, be aware that you may not like the result.*

> *Caution - If everything is a core value to you, then you'll have nothing to focus on.*

I desire to be more or have more....

Motivation, Drive, Achievement, Power, Ambition, Boldness, Authority, Leadership, Growth, Determination, Influence, Status, Success, Assertiveness, Decisiveness, Excellence, Results orientated, Strategic,

Adventurousness, Creativity, Curiosity, Freedom, Autonomy, Challenge, Exploration, Originality, Enthusiasm,

Beauty, Harmony, Proportion, Aesthetic Experience, Balance, Inner Peace, Restraint,

Challenges, Meaningful Work, Competency, Self-Respect, Accuracy, Competitiveness, Contribution, Reliable, Resourceful, Merit, Quality focused,

Citizenship, Community, Compassion, Kindness, Honesty, Security, Altruism, Belonging, Courtesy, Selflessness, Supportive, Usefulness, Patriotic, Equality, Unity, Nurturing,

Fame, Popularity, Recognition, Reputation, Respect, Responsibility, Service, Dependable, Disciplined,

Fun, Humour, Optimism, Cheerfulness, Excitement, Expressiveness, Spontaneity, Enjoyment,

Financial responsibility, Security, Wealth, Expertise, Preparedness, Stability, Timeliness, Order, Equity,

Knowledgeable, Truthful, Understanding, Wisdom, Honour, Esteem, Authenticity, Justice, Learning, Openness, Accountability, Clear minded, Improvement, Correctness, Diligence, Practical, Perfection, Tolerance,

Love, Mutual Affection, Family, Friendships, Contribution, Fairness, Cooperation, Loyalty, Trustworthiness, Fidelity, Sensitivity, Empathy,

Peace, Poise, Stability, Calmness, Contentment, Pleasure, Moral Disposition, Happiness, Fitness, Health, Traditionalism, Meditation,

Religion, Spirituality, Faith,

If you are able to live your life according to your own values, then generally you're doing well.

If you aren't then you'll need to change, either a little, or perhaps a lot.

> *Note - Your values will change overtime and changes in personal circumstances. I suggest you revisit this aspect of your life periodically.*

Protect yourself. Learn the laws that effect you, learn the ethics that pertain to you, and develop a set of morals that you feel comfortable with. Identify those values that you hold dear to who you are. Expand this list and be the master of who you are.

Do all of this now, as by doing so you'll enrich your life, and those people affected by your actions and beliefs. By teaching our children important values, the benefits of the law, ethical, and moral behaviour, we will help develop happier and more enlightened adults and thereby improve the future of the generations that follow.

Studying philosophy will help you better understand these concepts, and how to adopt them into your personality, thereby enriching your life and its meaning. There are many books available that focus on these topics.

> *Observation - Many religious faiths teach values that are beneficial to the individual, family, or group. You don't need to be religious to have values, but if you feel you are floundering, then participating in regular religious congregations may be beneficial for you.*

~ 20 ~

WHY IT'S GOOD TO FEEL PRIDE AND TO BE PROUD OF YOUR SKILLS AND ACHIEVEMENTS.

> *Quote - I'd rather be partly great than entirely useless. — Neal Shusterman*

> *Note - Your **Ability** is what you're capable of doing. Your **Motivation** determines what you do, and your **Attitude** determines how well you will do it. Aim to have all three of these in your skill sets.*

Having pride is the intense deep feeling of satisfaction or pleasure derived from a personal achievement. It can also be felt when a person who is close to you (such as a family member) completes a valued achievement.

Being proud is the intense deep feeling of satisfaction or pleasure derived from a personal achievement. It can also be felt when a person who is close to you (such as a family member) completes a valued achievement. Hang-on. Those are the same words I just used to explain pride.

A person can be proud or have pride but not do so in reverse. Pride is a noun and proud is an adjective. You can take pride in being proud.

So why am I talking about it in this book? Well, having too much pride or being too proud is regarded as a bad thing. Others will judge you harshly because of it and it may impact on your quality of enjoyment of life and your achievements.

The trick here is modesty and moderation. Having pride in one's work, artistic skill, athletic achievement, or other worthy endeavours, forms an important aspect of motivation. We enjoy the feeling, so we want more of it. When a person exhibits showy behaviour because of their achievements, they cross the line and become obnoxious to others who will proceed to alienate them. Humans will allow a high achiever their moment to bask in glory so long as it isn't prolonged beyond reason.

Note - A narcissist is a person who has a self-centred personality, with excessive interest in their own needs, excessive self-promotion of achievements, (real or imagined) with little or no regard for others or their feelings. They can be offended when challenged and when they occupy a position of authority or leadership, they can be very unfair and detrimental to others, particularly spouses and subordinates. Sometimes, the behaviour can be as a result of a medical disorder, but culturally, we'll believe it to be intentional and we'll disapprove of it.

Being told by someone who is significant to you that they are proud of you and your achievements can be very rewarding if done in moderation. Excessive adulation will rapidly dilute its value.

So, what does it mean to be too proud, and why is this labelled a bad thing to do? Simply, we all need help from time to time.

When we do, and help is offered, the polite thing to do is to accept graciously, but only after determining if there are any unreasonable conditions associated with that assistance. If rejected, and things get worse as a result of that rejection, the incumbent is seen as having stubborn pride, and therefore foolish for rejecting the assistance. An example of this is an unemployed person rejecting a job offer they see as beneath them. This becomes amplified when others are adversely affected by the stubbornness of one person.

Wounded pride is when someone's ego has been humiliated, real or imagined. The danger here is the counter actions taken are often disproportionate to the insult, making the situation worse and not better. If you feel wounded pride, it is best to take a step away from the problem, break it down into its components, ask yourselves the extent of your own contribution, determine the true damage, discuss the situation with a trusted other, find a positive way to get back on task. Focus on the solution, not the problem.

Stubborn pride is when the person is too short-sighted and insecure to respond to assistance even when it is clearly needed as it may hurt their feelings. Children exhibit this and constant parental capitulation can lead to a permanent undesirable character trait. The best solution I can offer is that you should present the evidence and allow it to be absorbed by the recipient in their own time. Be sure it is presented at a level they can understand, without being patronising.

> *Note - Pride has ancient origins as being evil and hence the confusion over it today. It is also known as a hubris and is considered to be the worst of the seven deadly sins. It is the opposite of humility.*

Pride has been associated with selfishness, shaming others, anger, greed, and the putting of one's own needs constantly before others. Hence its bad reputation.

Being proud, and having pride is a good thing, but keep it in its proper place.

> *Quote – Failure is not falling down; it is refusing to get back up.*
> *Stephan De Jonghe*

~ 21 ~

WHY WE SHOULD UNDERSTAND NEEDS, WANTS, AND HAVE TOO.

> *Quote - The average person needs only two things to become wealthy. 1) the knowledge of what to do, 2) the discipline to practice the things that need to be done. Noel Whittaker.*

The philosophical view on the difference between needs and wants, is that you should only acquire what you need in order to have a good life, with a little in reserve. Everything else is an excess.

However true that philosophy is, it isn't a popular point of view. Humans like to accumulate things or stuff. Particularly wealth. We love to see growth in assets and bank balances, and we even name them securities because they make us feel more secure. It gives meaning to many of us. It is their reason for getting up and doing things. They feel motivated by accumulation.

Growth as a child means getting taller, gaining skills, academic pursuits, sporting achievements, having friends, earning respect, and achieving independence.

Growth as an adult is about forming permanent relationships, increasing wealth, accumulating assets, gaining wisdom, improving skills, making life choices, pursuing interests and hobbies, being philanthropic, managing health and fitness, retiring with dignity, and dying peacefully.

So, why is need, have, and want, so important to understand? Why do we contemplate the possible outcomes?

Firstly, we should define them.

Need – (a) Something you require because it is essential or very important. (b) A necessity or obligation.
Example. (a) I need quality food, water, shelter, and safety to sustain my life. (b) I need to care for my family.

Have – (a) Something you own. (b) Something you wish on yourself as an outcome of an event. (c) Something you feel obligated to do or to obtain.
Example. (a) I have a car. (b) I hope I have a good time at the party. (c) I have to pay taxes.

Want – (a) A desire to possess something you may or may not need. (b) Something you'd like to do or achieve.
Example – (a) I want new shoes. (b) I want to learn to drive a car.

Often the same example can be used for all three words. I need to clean my home. (I can't find anything, and it smells bad) I have to clean my home. (My partner will punish me if I don't) I want to clean my home. (I'll feel better for doing it, after all it is my home). Wanting to clean your room makes the task easier and more enjoyable.

> *Observation – Many people get busy tidying their home in preparation for visitors, (especially true for parents and in-laws). Shouldn't they do the housework for their own benefit?*

Another example. I need to pay taxes. (Governments need the revenue to provide services to the community). I have to pay taxes. (It is the law and there are penalties for not doing so). I want to pay taxes. (It means I've earned the money, and that I'm doing well, and I like the society I live in, and that costs money, which is raised via taxation). Wanting to pay taxes makes taxation less of a burden.

Next example – I need to go to work. (It is where the money comes from). I have to go to work. (I'll get dismissed if I don't) I want to go to work. (It is where the money comes from, and I feel productive about earning it. I want to provide for my family, I want to acquire the things I desire, and I want to feel part of a team). Wanting to go to work makes it far easier to do so.

So, the lesson here on how to improve your life is to rethink your attitude towards need to have to and want to. Change your mind set from the things you need to do, and have to do, into being the things that you want to do. Add an emotional benefit to it. Own this attitude so that you hear yourself saying more often that I want to do this, as opposed to I need to do it, or have to do it. You'll become more productive and happier as a result.

As humans, our greatest priority is to firstly satisfy our needs. Those people that can't, often need outside assistance. Charities, and government agencies, are inundated with requests for help from people requiring assistance with obtaining basic needs. The tragedy comes from the high ratio of people who need assistance because they put their wants before their needs. Examples of this include gambling irresponsibly and trying to use it as a short-cut to accumulate wealth quickly and without having to earn it. A second example is when people are living beyond their means. Examine global credit card debt to understand this problem.

There are many victims who have been scammed and others who have been betrayed both financially and emotionally by a spouse, or another family member. Some people simply followed bad advice through ignorance, all in the misguided hope that it will work out all right, despite not having any trustworthy evidence to prove that it will do so.

Many people suffer temporary setbacks in their lifetime and genuinely need short term assistance to get them back to self-sufficiency. Many people lack skills on how to manage income, expenditure, set priorities, research opportunities and maximise their options. Hopefully, by reading this book they will gain some benefit in this area.

Despite being offered opportunity, training, and guidance, some people will never achieve independence from outside assistance. Some people are fortunate to live a society that will try to provide for people in those circumstances. Sadly, many do not.

~ 22 ~

THE DECISION-MAKING PROCESS.

People are essentially habit forming. We love routines and consistency. When we find a product we like, we stick to it. When we receive good service, we go back to them. When we've gone through the process and found a provider that meets or exceeds our expectations we use them again, even years later. We are also quick to tell others how much we like the product or how we appreciated their service. Consequently, we are also quick to judge harshly when we are dissatisfied, and with the use of social media, we have a ready platform to vent and share our thoughts with others.

How do we actually make the decision to buy a product or use a service? These are the steps we should be taking.

1. We identify a need or a want for something, or have the need brought to our attention by others. They include salespeople offering a solution or becoming better informed through advertising.
2. We research the variables and reach a conclusion from all the options. We consider brand, product features, suitability, reliability, reputation, and cost.

3. We perform a simple cost benefit evaluation and ask ourselves is this worth it?
4. We make a purchase decision and complete the transaction. We measure this process and determine if it was easy and simple, or we conclude it was too difficult and it should be avoided in the future.
5. We evaluate our decision and ask ourselves "was it fair?" This process will either justify our decision and we'll feel good about it, or we'll experience buyers' remorse and feel bad about it. We'll often share these feelings with others.
6. When we have repeated steps one through five several times for the same product or service and we have positively validated our decision, then this becomes our automatic buying and rebuying behaviour.
7. However, if the product changes, then we'll most likely restart the process. For example, changes to availability, brand, features, suitability, formulation, reliability, reputation, and price. This also includes changes to service satisfaction or changes to the staff of that service provider.

We humans are loyal to retailers, our banks, our doctors, dentists, and tradespeople. As long as they don't change and keep doing a good job then we generally keep going back to them. We say things like "If it isn't broken why risk change", and "I know what I like and I know who I trust".

Loyalty, trust, and imparting consumer confidence is important for humanity. We have so many aspects of life to consider and so by having confidence in products, retailers and service providers we use, is beneficial to our mental health.

Opportunity cost. This is when you forgo the benefit you might have received if you had chosen a different option. For example: You can't eat your cake and still have it. Decision making is complex and more often than not it is not choosing between doing or not doing, but deciding which of the known choices will bring about the best satisfaction, happiness, or reward.

It is also handy to understand the law of diminishing benefit. This is when a second item of the same thing has less value than having it the first time. For example: owning two copies of the same movie has almost no benefit, (unless the first one stops playing) whereas owning a second bar of gold, does.

~ 23 ~

THE END OF YOUR LIFE, AND THE END OF THIS BOOK.

> *Quote - I'm not as young as I used to be, but then I'm not as old as I'm going to be. Dik Brown*

If, during your old age, you can reflect on your life and say "I've lived a good, happy, and rewarding life" then you have done well. Having a high quality of life is more important than the quantity of life. Wanting to live longer should be about achieving more for yourself and for others. Living a life filled with regrets would be for me, the saddest outcome as I believe regrets should be avoided.

The toughest aspects of advanced aging are –

1. Loss of motivation.
2. Reduced dexterity.
3. Being patronised.
4. Being labelled as old, or too old.
5. Dementia.
6. Loss of a spouse or life partner.
7. Surrendering control over decision making.
8. Relinquishing a driver's licence.

9. Persistent, and often painful, debilitating health issues.
10. Financial stress.
11. Worry over the lack of the provisions made for your surviving spouse or life partner.
12. Worrying about the equitable provisions that you made in your Will or Testament. Having too little to pass on after your death.
13. Being put under emotional pressure from family members to do things you don't agree with or understand.
14. Missing the opportunity to make right past wrongs and making peace with troubled family members and friends.
15. Dying.

These stresses can be mitigated by proper preparation and provision in the years to leading up to advanced aging. Get trusted and professional help before you enter the advanced aging stage.

> *Tip - Treat elderly people the way you'd like to be treated when it's your turn to be old. Remember that your children are watching, and they are learning from your example.*

The concepts of Heaven and Hell were first devised thousands of years ago. In ancient Greek times they believed in an afterlife place called Hades, named after the mythical Greek God, who ruled it. It had three levels. The best level and one that all ancient Greeks aspired too, was known as Elysium, which is a Christian equivalent to Heaven. The middle level, where most ordinary souls ended up, was called Asphodel Gardens (After a flower common in the Mediterranean) and interestingly, there is no Christian equivalent. It was said to be a very simple place, offering little in the way of pleasure, but also no discomfort or pain. The worst level was called Tartarus and it is the equivalent of what Christians describe as Hell.

These mythical places still persist in our imaginations today and they still influence human behaviour. Is it that the promise of life after death, luxuriating in heaven, is only a bribe or incentive to better behaviour? Is it a positive religious belief that good behaviour in life will somehow be rewarded in the afterlife?

Is the torment of Hell, and the threat of damnation and eternal punishment for bad behaviour, as measured out by your peers, only the threat? Was it just about crowd control, and a way to mollify our potential disruptive behaviour? As humanity becomes more enlightened, shouldn't we need these measures less and less?

> *Music Quote - Some folks live with no reason; some folks die without warning. Alice Cooper 1975*

What troubles most of us about death is the actual process of dying. For some it is sudden, and the grief and remorse is felt by others. For many, the dying process is protracted, and often there is pain associated with their final stages of life. It is this process of actually dying, that is truly the worrying part.

Hopefully, when it is your turn, you will have the best medical support to see you through this process. Hopefully, you will be in the company of compassionate loved ones to assist you in your final days. Sadly, for some people, this isn't true.

> *Quote - Make sure before your dying day, that all of your faults die with you. - Seneca*

Love conquers all, hatred consumes all, and when all else fails, only hope remains.
The final word is always... death.

> *Tip - Before you die, remember that the way you behave in your latter years will be how others will remember you. It is great to be old, it means you've lived a long life, but do so with dignity and self-respect. Be kind, gracious, and appreciative to those people who care for you. Reflect on your happy memories and be grateful you had the opportunity to make them.*

Sadly, we've reached the end of this book, but it is not actually the end of learning. Make it your personal mission to do so.

There are many more topics I can write about to help you better understand and guide you through "Your Meaning of your Life". Let's get this book into circulation and when there is sufficient interest, I'll continue our journey together with a sequel.

Cheers
Stephan De Jonghe

ABOUT ME AS AN AUTHOR

> *Observation - Authors are quick to explain that you can't edit a blank page. Editing is different from creating, but it occupies the bulk of the author's time spent on the planned publication. Tweaking also heavily features in preparing the final version. A tweak is a minor improvement, and you feel good for doing it, but you also feel bad because you worry about how many more you could do.*

My name is Stephan De Jonghe, and I am an avid reader and writer. I started my writing journey as a playwright and I wrote four full-length comedies, and several one-act plays, which were performed before appreciative audiences.

They are, Death Warmed Up, Meals Warmed Up, Lovely Lobster Tale, The Culpeper Code, Free coffee for the driver, Life and a bottle of tomato sauce, Death of a Scotsman, and Hyp-no-me. For details about my plays visit https://www.taztix.com.au/stephan-jean-de-jonghe/.

I next turned my focus on writing a comedy titled "Follicle Farm – A novel Adventure" which was self-published in 2022. This book is now available from all major on-line book sellers. More details about "Follicle Farm – A novel Adventure" are at the end of this book and on the Follicle Farms website www.folliclefarm.com.au

> *Quote – Authors spend an inordinate amount of time editing their thoughts. Stephan De Jonghe*

This publication, "Your concise guide to the meaning of life," is the culmination of decades of research that I have done on how to live a great life.

I found gaps in what I read, and so I decided to write a self-help book to help others who may also feel they are missing some information on how to successfully enjoy their lives.

Whilst I'm not clinically qualified to professionally help people, I do have life experiences, and I'm willing to publicly share them for the potential benefit of readers. This book is meant to be a back-to-basics approach to understanding what about your own life has value to you.

> *Observation - I'm fascinated with my own psychological profile.*

I've spent the last 45 years working in the food industry in Perth, Western Australia. I have formal studies in Business Management and Sales and Marketing. My work skill sets include customer service, market research, new product development, sales and key account management, business reviews, sales team management, business plans, and heaps more.

During this time, I've met and dealt with a lot of very interesting people. Some have inspired me about what, and how, to live my life. Most have shown me what not to do.

Either way, I benefited.

I'm happily married to Deb, and we live in Perth, Western Australia, Australia.

FOLLICLE FARM

At the time of this book's publication, Follicle Farm is available in paperback or e-book form from...
AbeBooks - Germany
Amazon – Australia
Amazon - UK
Angus & Robertson Books - Australia
Barnes and Noble
Bokus (Sweden)
Book Depository – UK
Bookshop.org - USA
Booktopia
Buffalo Street Bookstore – Ithaca, New York
Donner - Nederland's
Dymocks - Australia
Fishpond – New Zealand
Good Reads
Kobo
Readings – Victoria, Australia.
SCRIBD – California, USA.
Walmart – Sacramento, USA
Waterstones – UK
National Library of Australia
State Library of Western Australia.

Welcome to Follicle Farm. Bobby is a Mitochondria, and he works as a humble Follicle Farmer. He, with millions of colleagues, is part of the amazing organisation dedicated to growing hair for the human male that they live inside of. Recently, Bobby made an important discovery when he learned how to reverse the effects of alopecia and greying hair. Now it's up to management to debate if they should use his technique.

Join Bobby as he travels the body, ably assisted by Banjo and Skip, as he meets and deals with other human cells in various systems throughout the body. Bobby quickly learns there is more to management than just servicing the body's needs. Cliques, quirks, politics, unions, and hidden agendas, all thrive in Bobby's world.

You'll share in his adventure of personal growth as he encourages other Follicle Farmers to utilise best-practices in growing quality hair. Follicle Farm is comic and imaginative insight into organisational structure and behaviour of the trillions of cells that make up the microscopic world of every living person. It reveals how cells within the human body really think and how they, mostly, work well together. This is Bobby's story....

www.folliclefarm.com.au

www.ingramcontent.com/pod-product-compliance
Lightning Source LLC
Chambersburg PA
CBHW070307010526
44107CB00056B/2520